BUILDING HANDWRITING SKILLS

in dyslexic children

Edited by John I. Arena

ACADEMIC THERAPY PUBLICATIONS

San Rafael, California 94901

Academic Therapy Publications
P.O. Box 899
1539 Fourth Street
San Rafael, California 94901

Books, tests, and materials
for and about the learning disabled

Library of Congress
Catalog Number: 70-134384

The cover and some of the handwriting samples through
the courtesy of Norma Banas, I. H. Wills and the
children at Educational Guidance Services, Miami.

First printing: 1970
Second printing: 1972
Third printing: 1974
Fourth printing: 1976

Printed in the United States of America

Introduction

NO ONE could even begin to estimate the number of adults who are hampered by the inability to write legibly and easily. Poor handwriting, often a graphic symptom of learning disorders, plagues children, their parents, and their teachers from the first grade through college and beyond. It limits academic expression, inhibits spontaneous productivity, and affects communication. It is a disabling nuisance that creative and productive people can ill afford.

Poor handwriting comes packaged in many forms. It may be tight, jagged, or squeezed; it may be improperly spaced or disorganized; it may be slanted uphill, downhill, or roller-coastery; it may be miniscule or gargantuan — or it may be simply an indescribable scrawl.

It would seem obvious that in the majority of instances the time-hallowed procedure of circling poor handwriting with red pencil simply does not produce the desired results. In my early teaching days, as so many others have done before and since — and with every honorable intention in the world — I had a small group of children come to school before class each day to practice writing on the chalkboard or at their desks, hoping, I imagine, that something quite marvelous would happen if they did it over and over again. In spite of my warm support and continued encouragement, at the end of the year I could discern little real improvement in the child's handwriting or in the ease with which he tried to execute the forms.

In addition to the "repetition" approach, three other methods have had popular appeal. One is the he'll-outgrow-it; give-him-time method. Another is the he-could-do-better; insist-on-it approach. The third is the just-show-him-how; he'll-catch-on technique. While these approaches may work in some few cases, they unfortunately fail for the staggering majority of children who are having trouble learning to write. These youngsters can be described as scrawling their way through school, a puzzle to busy teachers with already heavy teaching responsibilities. The result is that the extent of remedial assistance is often continual admonishments to "Please take greater pains to turn in neater papers."

We know how important and rewarding it is for the child to learn to produce clear, consistent, and legible handwriting. It would seem that the mistake so often made in the past is that we take it for granted that children *should* and *could* achieve this goal that it becomes difficult to understand why they *don't*.

The fact that so many young people are still unable to write well when they graduate from high school indicates that the problem is not self-correcting with the passage of time. We know also that most children admire fine handwriting and are proud when they see improvement in their own. They have a natural need and desire to communicate. We have all seen children struggling valiantly to form letters and words correctly so that they say something and can be read by others. Motivation alone, then, is not the answer.

It seems our failure has been that we have not seen handwriting skill as but a part of the whole child. We have tended incorrectly to isolate it as a separate phenomenon. As a result we have treated it as such by "piece-mealing" the child and concentrating on training only his hands. Even worse, we have found labels to explain the child's lack of progress and to rationalize our own inability to help him, rather than using this as a starting point to begin training his sensory and motor functions to respond in a more controlled and efficient manner.

We have failed to fully realize the impact of deep-rooted developmental, maturational, perceptual, emotional, and socio-cultural forces and their vital involvement in the child's ability or nonability to produce the graphic form of handwriting. We have too often assumed "readiness" at a particular chronological age level when not fully understanding what developmental states were needed and whether or not this particular child had progressed in vital areas to that extent.

As specialists from all fields allied and related to the identification, diagnosis, and remediation of learning disabilities, we must be concerned with handwriting because it is one of the communication skills and has a domain of consequence commensurate with the tools of reading, spelling, speaking, and listening.

T HE MAJORITY of the articles appearing in this collection originally appeared in the Fall 1968 issue of *Academic Therapy* — an issue devoted entirely to this problem. The demand for copies was so great that the supply was almost immediately depleted. Two years later the orders were still arriving, demonstrating the continuing need for this material.

We are indebted to all the authors who generously agreed to have their papers included in this collection. Grateful appreciation is extended to Dr. Milton Eger, editor of the *Journal of the American Optometric Association*, and to the *South African Journal of Occupational Therapy*, for permission to include the articles by Dr. Kahn and Mrs. Harrison, which initially appeared in their journals.

The authors, in each case, describe what they have found to be helpful. No attempt has been made to make this collection into a *method*; consequently there are points of diversification as well as points of agreement. This is what we feel makes the collection broad and applicable to many situations and settings. It is hoped that what is offered here will be tried, explored, varied, expanded, and creatively used to help the children — our ultimate goal.

J. I. A.

CONTENTS

The Brain-Damaged Child and Writing Problems

Enid M. Harrison

A NY CHILD without brain damage can have a writing problem. This may be due to one or more of the following factors:

- Physical disability.
- Defective eyesight.
- Hand dominance not established.
- Emotional problems.
- Lag in the stages of perceptual development as in the slow-learning child.
- Retardation.

In a class of cerebral-palsied children, where we know there is brain damage, all the factors mentioned above may well be present, and if the teacher is to find the cause of the problem she must have a clear picture of the child as a "whole." She will be guided in this assessment of the child by a team of workers — pediatrician, neurologist, ophthalmologist, orthopedic surgeon, psychologist, speech therapist, occupational therapist, physiotherapist, and social worker.

In this article, however, it is intended to exclude the above listed factors and to discuss writing problems resulting from lack of readiness skills due to faulty integration and interpretation of sensations — sensory, motor, and proprioceptive — within the brain; that is, specific problems caused by disabilities in specific areas of perception.

The Neurological Writing Problem.

W HEN WORKING with brain-damaged children, it is most important to know that:

- Some children may have no learning problems; others may have one or two or many.
- These problems may exist to a lesser or greater degree.
- The perceptual disability, resulting in the same problem, may be different in each child.
- The problem may be due to one or a combination of perceptual disabilities.

As a result, no two of these children are ever the same and the test included in this article should enable the teacher/therapist to detect the exact nature of each child's perceptual disability. There are also children with minimal brain damage, but no physical handicap, who have the same neurological learning problems as the cerebral-palsied child.

It is generally accepted that perceptual development, upon which learn-

1

ing readiness skills are based, appears to be at its maximum between the ages of two and one-half and seven and one-half years. It is also accepted that the different perceptual abilities develop independently of each other, and this is clearly seen in psychological test results of the brain-damaged child where there can be considerable discrepancy in the various spheres of ability. For example:

• A child may read well but have a writing problem.

• A child may be able to perceive position in space but be unable to see the relationship of one part to another.

After the age of seven and one-half years (mental age), reasoning processes become progressively more important than perceptual development, and this factor is most important in planning a remedial program for the child of average or above-average intelligence.

AT THE Forest Town School for Cerebral Palsied Children, very young babies are treated as out-patients, and children between the ages of two to three years are admitted to the Nursery School where training and further assessment, through observation of the child, is continued. This early assessment of the child's abilities and disabilities may well indicate later learning problems, as well as providing a basis for a training program. The stages of perceptual development in the normal child must always be kept in mind.

In order to be able diagnostically to use the test given in this article and to plan a remedial program in which the child's abilities will be used to overcome his disabilities, the teacher/therapist must have some knowledge of how perception develops through integration and interpretation of all the sensations.

In order for a child to be able to write, the following skills are necessary:

• He must be able to copy shapes; that is, to draw.

• He must be able to position these shapes correctly.

• He must be able to reproduce shapes.

In order to achieve these skills the child must have the following abilities:

I. *Visual Perception.* The ability to recognize objects, pictures, parts of a whole, and to discriminate.

II. *Visuo-Spatial Relationships.* The ability to perceive position in space; to judge size, distance, etc.; to be able to analyze, perceive relationships and integrate (synthesize) the following:

• The parts of the contour lines of a whole; for example, a square.

• The parts of a whole, for example, the letter K; a house made of a square, triangle (roof), and a chimney.

• The parts within a whole; for example, a mosaic. Also to perceive the relationship of one object to another, as in a picture.

III. *Visuo-Motor Ability.* The ability to manipulate spatial relationships; for example, to construct what has been perceived.

IV. *Eye-Hand Coordination.* The ability to reproduce (draw) what has been perceived.

V. *Recall.* The ability to recall and reproduce what has been perceived.

Below are given case histories to illustrate the following:

• How lack of one or more of the above abilities causes a writing problem.

• That if there is inability to perceive correctly in Section I (that is, there is faulty "input" or agnosia), there will be inability to reproduce correctly.

• That even if there are no "input" problems in Section I but there is faulty "input" in Section II, there will be an inability to reproduce correctly.

• That if there is no "input" problem, but there is an inability to reproduce correctly, then there is an "output" problem, or apraxia (the inability to carry out the motor act necessary for reproducing what is perceived), described in Sections III and IV.

Case Histories.[1]

Janey, age seven, could recognize an object, but could not recognize the picture of that object. She could not perceive the "form" or picture against a background. It took two years to teach her to write and read. (This was in 1954, when very little was known about dealing with these problems.) Even after two years, the problem still existed, as shown in Illustration 1. The child's first attempt to copy this particular pattern shows how she saw the background and not the letter *O*.

Illustration 1.

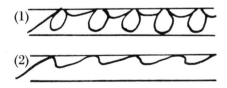

[1] The names used in the case histories are, of course, fictional.

[2] In all illustrations that follow, (1) is the teacher's drawing or the writing pattern, (2) is the child's copy.

Billy could recognize and match pictures and shapes — for example, squares, triangles, and circles — but could not recognize parts of a whole. As an example, in a picture of a man holding an umbrella under his arm, Billy could not recognize the umbrella because he could not see it as a whole. Also, he could not perceive a square as made up of parts, and therefore he could not reproduce its contour lines. At this stage (age seven), he was very keen on flowers and produced some excellent drawings of these done with crayons. This he was able to do because shape discrimination was good; he could perceive position in space and see the relationship of one whole to another. The flowers and the leaves on a stem were *drawn as shapes.* There were no outlines drawn, no separate petals making a flower, just the shape of the whole flower.

Fred had no "input" problems in Section I. In Section II, visuo-spatial relationships, his only disability was in determining right and left, so his only problem in writing was one of reversals. He wrote *d*'s, *b*'s, and *p*'s incorrectly and reversed the *S* and the number 3.

Susan had no "input" problems in Section I, but in Section II she could not determine right or left; nor could she perceive differences in position of objects at all. To her, pictures of baskets, two with handles to the top and the third upside down with the handle to the bottom, were exactly the same. Learning to write, therefore, was indeed a problem. Not only were there reversals, but an *n* was, to her, the same as *u* and *p* could be written like a *b*. After learning to make letters, she still did mirror writing and sometimes wrote from right to left — for example, she would write *mother* as *rehtom.*

Danny had problems in Section II. He could determine left and right, but he could not perceive position in space. Illustration 2 demonstrates his problem.

Illustration 2.

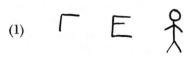

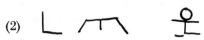

Danny could not see that his drawings were incorrect.

The only problem for Phil was one of poor judgment, resulting in an inability to space words, organize written work, and see relative sizes of letters. For example, he would write *mothers* as shown in Illustration 3 even if there were guiding lines.

Illustration 3.

(1)   mothers

(2) 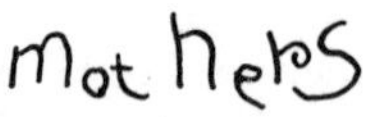   Mothers

Betty had no problems in Section I, and in Section II she could determine right and left, perceive position, analyze, see the relationship of one part to another in a whole, and she could integrate; but she could not position the parts correctly when constructing or drawing. For her drawing of the letter *K*, see Illustration 4. She could see the copy was incorrect, and when working with sticks or plasticine would, with much trial and error, push the pieces until they were in the correct position.

Illustration 4.

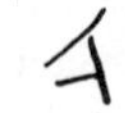

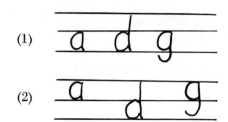

Betty also had difficulty in placing one object in correct relationship to another as shown in the illustration. (By this time she had learned to write the letters.) (See also Illustration 6.)

Carol had no problems in Section I, and in Section II she could determine right and left, perceive position, and analyze; but she could not see the relationship of one part to another. See her drawing of the letter *K* in Illustration 5.

Illustration 5.

(1)   K   (2) 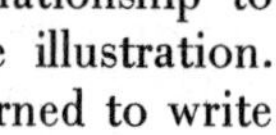 | \ ⟋

Anne had no problems in Section I, and in Section II she could determine right and left, perceive position, analyze, see the relationship of one part to another; but she could not relate them when constructing or drawing. Illustration 6 demonstrates her problem. (Note also Betty's interpretation of the original pattern.)

Illustration 6.

(1)

(2)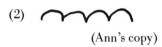

(Ann's copy)

(3)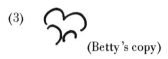

(Betty's copy)

Anne was also unable to place one object in relationship to another as illustrated in Betty's drawing of letters placed in lines. (Illustration 4.)

Brian had no problems in Section I, and in Section II could determine right and left, perceive position, analyze, see relationship, but could not perceive the integrated form and so drew a square. (See Illustration 7.)

Illustration 7.

(1) 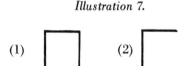 (2)

Patty had no "input" problems in either Section I or II, and she could copy any drawing. Visual memory was good, and she could easily recall a variety of objects seen; but she could not recall even a simple drawing. She could not remember the shape or the "pattern," so she could not write without a copy. Even after she had learned to write the letters without a copy, there were often reversals. This was not due to a right and left

inability, but because she could not recall the picture of the letter.

Jeff had no "input" problems in Section I, and in Section II he could perceive position, determine left and right, and could analyze and synthesize; but he could not see the relationship of one object to another at all. Because of body schema loss, he was unable to orientate himself in space and could not dress himself. He still cannot place his arm to put it into his jacket sleeve. It took years to teach him to form the letters because of this gross apraxia. He cannot organize written work, and still has difficulty in writing words with spaces in between. He cannot even place letters on a line. His inability to see the relationship of one object to another is clearly illustrated in a recent drawing of a vase containing flowers. He drew a vase and the flowers were drawn on the vase.

Assessment of the Child.

DURING the test, it is important to note the child's approach to a task, his ability to organize, concentration span, distractibility, and how he reacts in different situations; for example, when he is left to work on his own at matching pairs of cards, and when the teacher/therapist takes part by presenting the card so that the child can indicate the "odd" picture within a series of pictures. The test can still further be used to note the child's ability to benefit from suggestions as to how to improve his performance. For example, if the child has failed an item or found it difficult, demonstrate how he can perhaps use touch in discriminating shape, or how language can be used to interpret and/or

5

crystalize what is seen. Then, on the next item, note if and how he uses and benefits from the suggestions. The above information will be invaluable as a guide to the teacher/therapist when planning a remedial program for the child.

If the assessment is to be a true reflection of the child's potential, first make contact with the child and gain his confidence and interest. Also, make sure that the child understands what is expected of him in the different items so that the test situation does not become a "fearful" one, but rather a series of games which are fun.

THE TEST

THE TEST is divided into five sections already briefly discussed in this article. Where practicable, one example of each type of test material will be described and the teacher/therapist can then formulate the necessary extra apparatus. In the section on visuo-spatial relationships, descriptions of many of the pictures used to test the child's ability to perceive would be inadequate. Therefore, in these instances, it is intended instead to describe items in the section on visuo-motor ability to test the child's ability to manipulate spatial relationships and from these to assess his ability to analyze and perceive form as an integrated whole. These deductions can be made when the child constructs a shape and then compares it with the copy. For example, if the child's copy is incorrect and he cannot perceive this, then the problem is one of "input." If, however, the child can perceive that his copy is incorrect, the problem is one of "output."

I. VISUAL PERCEPTION.
  A. Recognition.
    1. Objects: doll, car, dog, ball, bottle, etc.

2. Pictures of these objects. (One drawing on a page.)
  a. In color.
  b. In outline.

B. Matching.
  1. Object and picture (as used in A).
  2. Pairs of picture cards; for example:
    a. Green balls; yellow balls; dolls with red jackets; dolls with blue jackets; cars with wheels outlined in red; cars with wheels outlined in green.
    b. Houses without a chimney, etc.
  3. Three-dimensional objects (two of each).
  4. Two-dimensional objects (two of each); for example, a square, triangle, circle, cotton reel.
  5. Drawing of above in outline (two of each).
  6. Fitting the above two-dimensional objects into correct spaces (Montessori form board).
  7. Fitting three-dimensional objects (as above) into correct spaces (for example, postbox).
  8. Finding the "odd" picture. (Four or five pictures on one card; for example, four identical and one odd picture.) Illustrations might be plants with a flower and one without, or rabbits with both ears and one with an ear missing, etc.

C. Part-Whole Ability. (Recognition of a whole from a part.)
  1. Objects: for example, expose part of a doll or have half a

doll, car, bottle, etc., and the child names the object.

2. Pictures: child to name objects.
   a. Pictures of parts of the objects used in C-1; for example, half a bottle.
   b. Picture of the top and bottom parts of a bottle with the middle missing.

D. Figure – Background.

1. Pairs of picture cards: drawings to be in outline against different backgrounds; for example, a cup with a background of crosses on one card and on the other a background of wavy lines; a car with the same backgrounds as for the cup. (Does the child match the form seen against the background or does he match the backgrounds?)

2. Picture cards (three of each); for example, white square against a white background, a white square with contour lines in black against a white background, etc.

3. Drawings of a square, triangle, and circle on one card with a background of lines forming loops, etc. (The child is shown a two-dimensional square, triangle, circle and asked to find these shapes on the card.)

4. Drawings of a square, triangle, and a circle in outline superimposed one on the other.

   The child is shown a picture of, for example, the square in outline and is asked to find the shape on the card.

E. Form Constancy. (The ability to recognize shape in different colors, sizes, positions, etc.)

1. Objects: Place the following articles on the table and ask the child to match according to shape: clock, ring, ball, saucer, square box, toy table, toy chair, square picture frame.

2. Drawings on a card: for example, a square drawn inside another square, but at a different angle, a red square, a square with wavy lines inside.

   The child is shown the drawing of a square and is asked to indicate the squares on the card.

II. VISUO-SPATIAL RELATIONSHIPS.

A. The ability to discriminate, that is, perceive likenesses and differences in position. (Finding the "odd" picture on one card.)

1. Right-left discrimination.

   Pictures of people facing right and one facing left; curves to the right and one facing left; pictures of *d*'s and one *b*, etc.

2. *Up* and *down* discrimination.

   Pictures of baskets with handles to the top and one basket upside down with handle to the bottom; tables upside down and one right side up; pictures of *u*'s and one *n*, etc.

3. Direction.

   Make up cards, using identical and one odd picture on a card: lamp posts standing up, lying down, upside down, slanting up to the right and up to the left, slanting down to the left and to the right (lamp posts upside down).

B. Ability to judge size, length, height, distance. (Pairs of cards to be matched.)
1. Size: Pictures of small balls, big balls, small squares, big squares, small chairs, big chairs, etc.
2. Length: Pictures of long trains, short trains, long sticks, short sticks, etc.
3. Height: Pictures of tall men, short men, tall buildings, low buildings, etc.
4. Distance: Pictures of objects close together, far apart, etc.

C. Ability to analyze, perceive the relationship of one part to another and to synthesize.
1. Contour lines of a whole; for example, a square.
2. Parts of a whole; for example, a cat.
3. Parts within a whole; for example, a mosaic.

(Pictures on one card — identical drawings and one "odd.")

For 1 and 3 of Section C, geometric drawings are used. In 2 use, for example, a cat drawn as follows: small circle for head, big circle for body, curved line for tail; whiskers (three on each side) are drawn with the middle whisker straight out, the top one slanting up, the bottom one slanting down. On the card have identical pictures of cats, but on the odd one have the tail curved to the left if the other pictures have the tails curved to the right, and the direction of the whiskers different from the others.

D. Ability to perceive relationship of one object to another. (Pairs of cards to be matched.)

Picture with the sun in the top left corner, house in the middle, cat next to the house, tree in the right-hand bottom corner and a bird flying over the tree; the other picture with the sun, house, and tree in the same position, but with the cat under the tree and the bird flying over the house. The pictures are made up of circles placed in different positions.

III. VISUO-MOTOR ABILITY.

Ability to manipulate spatial relationships.

A. Placing objects in position. Having cutouts of pictures used in Section II-A (1, 2, and 3), and let the child place these in the same positions as those on the cards which were used. Note carefully whether the child is able to place the cutouts correctly without using the trial and error method.

B. Constructing what is perceived.

For constructing, use any of the following: key-way sticks (all the same length and in different colors), plasticine, straight and curved pieces of feltex in different sizes and colors (use the flannel board), straight and curved pieces of cardboard in different sizes and colors.
1. Contour lines of a whole.

Figures to be copied must be graded in difficulty. For example, a square, a triangle, a semicircle, figure made up of curves to the top left, right, and bottom, geometric figures made up of curves and straight lines.
a. Use different colors for the parts of the contour lines.

b. Use all the same color for the contour lines.

2. Parts of a whole.

Let the child construct a manikin, house, and a cat as in Section II-C (2).

Use geometric shapes, for example, circles, semicircles, triangles, squares, diamonds, rectangles, etc., to build a whole as in a mosaic. Figures to be graded in difficulty.

Note: Pictures or constructed figure, for the child to copy, must not be drawn or made in front of the child.

C. Placing objects in relation to each other.

Have cutouts of objects used in pictures as in Section II-D, and let the child construct the pictures with the cutouts.

IV. HAND-EYE COORDINATION.

This indicates the ability to follow eye movement with the hand and so draw what is perceived; also to initiate and stop movement.

A. Have straight and curved lines leading from one picture to another. For example, draw a dog with a straight line leading to a cat, a curved line leading from the cat to a mouse, and a straight line slanting up to the left leading from the mouse to its "hole." The child follows these lines, using a colored pencil.

B. Let the child copy one of the geometric designs used in Section II-B (1).

V. RECALL.

In A, memory recall is tested, whereas in B, C, and D the child's ability to visualize is tested.

A. Place objects on the table; for example, a doll, square, spoon, pencil, chair, brush. Remove the objects and ask the child to recall what he saw.

B. Place the objects in a row; for example, a square, triangle, circle, triangle, and a line straight up. Remove the objects and have the child draw or reconstruct what was perceived.

C. Construct a geometric figure in front of the child, remove the copy, and have the child construct the same figure.

D. Show the child a geometric figure (already constructed or drawn), remove the copy, and have the child construct the figure.

Remedial Teaching.

THE TEST will enable the teacher/ therapist to find out what is causing the child to have a writing problem, but in order to help the child overcome this problem, it is necessary to have a knowledge of how perception develops through integration and interpretation of all sensations — sensory, motor, and proprioceptive.

REFERENCES

Abercrombie, M. J. L. "Perceptual and Visuo-Motor Disorders in Cerebral Palsy," *Clinics in Developmental Medicine,* No. 11 (1964).

Berges, J., and I. Lezine. "The Imitation of Gestures," *Clinics in Developmental Medicine,* No. 18 (1965).

Frostig, Marianne, and David Horne. *The Frostig Program for the Development of Visual Perception.* Chicago: Follett, 1964.

Kephart, N. C. *The Slow Learner in the Classroom.* Columbus, Ohio: Charles E. Merrill, 1960.

Learning to read is like
learning to walk.
Its' harder to read
than it is to talk
I must learn to read
what I'm able to say
Or, I'll never be able
to earn a good pay

by Richard
8th grade

Teaching Beginning Writing

Charlotte E. Larson

VISUAL-PERCEPTUAL problems, neuro-motor deficiencies, space-perceptual lacks, background-foreground confusions, and body-concept difficulties will affect beginning writing. Many children who are known as children with severe learning disabilities have the above problems either separately or in combination.

In our special education program, we have no curriculum *per se,* nor do we have a one-way methodology for beginning handwriting. Our philosophy is to diagnose the needs of each child then plan the curriculum to meet those needs. The primary goals are (1) legible handwriting to be used as an aid in spelling and reading, and (2) written communication. Secondary to this will be the effect that learning to write has on training in the above-mentioned areas of deficit.

"Writing is a valuable and effective means of developing visuo-motor perception."[1] Writing, therefore, is a very essential skill and the readiness and beginning writing methods are especially important in training the child

who has an impairment of perceptive, expressive, or integrative functions. Beginning writing, in the "drawing" stage, may be structured if needed to compensate for (1) poor physical-motor function, (2) visuo-motor perceptual lacks, (3) background-foreground difficulties, and (4) spatial errors.

Heavy colored lines delineating the space to be written in for tall, small, and long letters will eliminate the background-foreground confusion caused by a sheet of paper with thirty blue lines all evenly spaced. A child who cannot stop at a colored line may need a frame made of cardboard so that as he hits the top or bottom colored line, the frame acts as a barrier and he has to stop.

Spatial errors leading to confusion of the direction in which lines extend in relation to the body may be aided by using arrows that are colored green (go) and red (stop), or the letter X for letters that start in space.

CURSIVE WRITING is recommended for a child who has many of the before-mentioned problems. All the lower-case letters start at the same line and never have to start

---

[1] A. A. Strauss and L. E. Lehtinen, *Psychopathology and Education of the Brain-Injured Child* (New York: Grune and Stratton, 1947).

out in space. Words, even though the spaces between the letters are irregular, hold together. If space between words is very small, there is still a separation between them. There is a rhythm, continuity, and wholeness to cursive.

Manuscript writing is done with straight lines, circles, and half-circles. Some letters are made with many parts and start at different places in space. The letters may look like disconnected strokes or loops if the child is not skillful in connecting them. Each letter must be separated by space and each word by a larger space. If space perception is poor then letters may become parts of other words.

T hec ati sont heb ox.

If the above sentence were in script and spaced exactly as above, it would still convey the meaning of the sentence.

Words, though close together, are still separated and letters spaced close or far apart still stay together with the connecting line.

Again, the kind of writing to be taught depends on the individual and the circumstances. If he has none or few of the above problems and he is in a first grade where all of his classmates write in manuscript, he should do so too.

THE FOLLOWING outline is given by Dr. L. E. Lehtinen in an unpublished paper on writing.[2]

---

[2]Laura E. Lehtinen, "Writing: Teaching Approaches to Establish Skills in Different Areas on Varying Levels." (Unpublished paper.)

I. Readiness (perceptuo-motor).
  A. Activities using gross motor arm movements.
  B. Activities with pencil, crayon, or felt pens using finer movements.
  C. Specific approaches.
II. Beginning writing (duplicating letter forms).
III. Beginning writing (spatial organization).
IV. Beginning writing (combining elements).
V. Relating cursive writing to print.
VI. Relating writing to speech: associating letters and speech sounds.
VII. Translating meaningful verbal patterns into written form.
VIII. Functional writing communication.

Since this article is on the teaching of beginning writing, we will go through only the first four steps of the above outline.

I. Readiness: Perceptuo-Motor.

IN WRITING readiness, tasks which promote the coordination of vision with the movements of the body or parts of the body should be used extensively. Building up the kinesthetic sense, which pertains to motor acts and is the perception or consciousness of one's own muscular movements, is of great importance in pre-writing.

We have no space receptor. Our body is the axis of our space world and all knowledge regarding space must be learned through experimentation.

The child should do a variety of gross muscular movements, such as *up, down, out, back, forward, backward, left to right, diagonal,* and *up and down* on the same line. This last movement is necessary when you make certain letters, such as *d, h, m,* etc. Both arms should do the movement simultaneously. Verbalization should be encouraged if there is a problem. Verbalization will help to reinforce the direction of the movement.

With a piece of chalk in each hand, the child should draw circles (1) first going upward and out, (2) then in the opposite direction – going upward and in, and starting at a distance away from the body. Draw a house or a garage on the blackboard directly in front of the child's eyes and have him take a piece of chalk in each hand and reach out as far as he can and draw lines which end in the house.

Have the child, using the preferred hand, draw the following from one side of the blackboard all the way across to the other side:

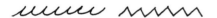

Besides the movement of the eyes and arm, he must also move his body by moving his feet across a space. Following are other suggested exercises:

The teacher and the child stand together at the blackboard. The teacher places a dot on the board designating the starting point. As the child places his chalk on the dot, the teacher makes another dot, saying, "Hit this."

Following each new dot, the child moves the chalk up, down, left, right, and diagonal (crossing the midline of the body). The teacher also places dots in strategic places, forcing the child to cross over lines.

Another suggested exercise is for the teacher to place a line of dots in a row and have the child go over, under, over, under:

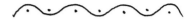

Still using large patterns, have the child trace, with different colored chalk, over white or yellow chalk patterns made by the teacher:

/ + X O ∩ ∪ − |

Using green for "start" or "go" and red for "stop," make dots either on large paper or the blackboard for vertical, horizontal, and diagonal lines. It is best to have the green dot at the bottom and the red at the top, as later the child will learn that all the letters (lower case) begin at the bottom green line.

AFTER the chalkboard activities, which are exercises involving gross arm movements, the child can begin to work with crayon or pencil, which will require finer movements. Have him start by tracing through onion skin. A good grade of onion skin or tracing paper should be used. This is placed over a pattern of brightly colored directional lines, patterns, drawings, or forms made with colored marking pens. For some children, it might be best to begin with a one-fourth sheet of work and then progress to a half then a whole sheet.

The pattern and tracing sheet should be thumbtacked to a board. If the child's motor needs require it, the board may be C-clamped to the desk. Using different colors for the patterns helps to hold the child's attention to completion of the project.

After tracing, have the child reproduce the patterns within a structured space, such as a one-inch or a two-inch space. The teacher may draw thick boundary lines on the paper.

13

If these lines do not provide sufficient structure for the child, a sheet of heavy cardboard, the size of the sheet of paper, should be cut so as to have two-inch spaces across the cardboard. This is tacked over the writing paper to enable the child to stay within the lines. From the patterns, he should be asked to copy the same sets he has just traced. This stage of the program includes a greater variety of directional lines, patterns, forms ,and drawings than the child has worked with before.

Colors, arrows, X's, or dots should be used to designate directions, for highlighting common errors or parts usually left out (such as the *three* humps in the *m*), and for stopping and starting points.

Writing in a clay pan with a stylus or in a sand pan with a finger will help reinforce the pattern both kinesthetically and tactually. The movement and directionality must be specifically patterned and closely supervised by the teacher so the child does not practice and reinforce errors.

II. Beginning Writing.
(Duplicating Letter Forms.)

IN BEGINNING writing we duplicate the letter forms. The correct motor pattern of the letter must be recalled when it is seen or when its name or sound is heard. The letters that go away from the body are taught first. There are two reasons for this procedure: movement away from the body is more easily controlled and these letter sounds are more easily differentiated.

The letter is made (with the preferred hand) in the air, on the chalkboard, and then on a large sheet of unlined paper. Next it is written on structured paper.

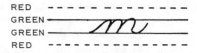

The letters all start with the bottom green line. Most of the letters stay between the green lines, but we let *t, l, j, h, k,* and *b* go to the top red line and we let *z, y, j, p, g,* and *q* go to the bottom red line. We let *f* go to the top red line and to the bottom red line, but it must tie at the bottom green line.

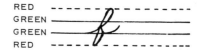

We use a simplified alphabet. The letter *d* goes up to the top line and down on the same line. We do not use the loop in either the *d* or the *p*. If these letters are formed with a loop and the loop is not closed, *d* may easily become *cl* and the letter *p*, if drawn out, may look like *j*.

Colors can be used to differentiate visual differences in letters such as *l, k, b,* and *h*, by making the one part of each letter that is alike in the same color, and making the part which is different in a second color. The letter *m*, which has three "over the hills" and a "tail," can be made in four colors — one for each part. The child makes it with a chalk or pencil in one color only so that the gestalt or total form, as he writes it, is not broken. He sees the visual difference of the parts as they are in color, but the motor pattern is not interrupted if he does not use different colors.

As he writes the letters, the child says the sound of the letter orally so as to connect the auditory with the visuo-motor learnings.

Beginning letters should be taught first and then the derived letters. For example, *l* is learned, with its straight down stroke to the bottom green line, then *h* is learned. The letter *h* is a derived letter because it has the same first two parts, and only the "hump" is different.

Beginning Letters	Derived Letters
m n	*x z v y*
t i u w r s	*j p*
l e	*h b k f*
a c d o	*g q*

III. Beginning Writing. (Spatial Organization.)

WHEN THE motor patterns of the letters have been learned, then the child can be expected to put them in the right space. Again, the size of the space to be used will depend on the needs of the individual child. Many children may have to have wide colored lines for demarcation, or a wide space in which to write the letters. Any structure should be provided that will allow the individual to experience success.

The writing space of the control paper has red lines at the top and bottom and green lines for the two middle lines.[3] There are four lines and three spaces so there is a designated line for both the tall and the long letters to touch.

At this stage, children should be able to make letters from copy. The left-handed child may need his copy at the top of the paper so he does not cover up the sample as he writes.

---

[3]This control paper may be obtained from DLM Company, 3505 North Ashland Avenue, Chicago, Illinois 60657.

IV. Beginning Writing. (Combining Elements.)

AS THE CHILD proceeds with writing, he should be able to write two to three different letters on a line so he can change motor patterns easily. Next, the child should make two letters joined. Since he sounds the letters orally, it is a good idea to use two letters that make a word, such as *in, it, is, up, on, as,* or *an.* By naming the *e* and the *o* (or giving them the long sound), the following may be written: *me, he, be, we, or, go, so,* and *no.*

Most of the connecting lines of letters are at the line, but those that are not must be taught. Examples are letters that have tails at the top, such as *o, v,* or *w;* or the *b,* which is joined at the middle. Where errors are made, color should be used to call attention to the placement of the connecting line.

Beginning writing has been taught by use of a very structured plan and adherence to the rules is required of the student. In writing capitals, for example, we begin by discussing the need for them. They are used to begin a person's name, for the first letter in a sentence, for names of cities, days, months, etc. In order to show this, we must make the first letter look different. The child may have a choice in the way he makes the capital; it must be different looking, but the need must come first.

If a child is having difficulty, he may choose the upper-case printed letter. This is accepted for the time being, but the child is encouraged to experiment and practice different capitals, such as *f, t, b,* and *r.* He is shown that capital letters can start out with a loop or a cane: *ℐ.* If the loop causes problems, a modified cane may be used: *ꜱ* . This approach makes youngsters less rigid and reinforces the

15

fact that letters may be of different sizes, shapes, and patterns yet still be the designated letter.

Visuo-motor problems, space-perceptual deficiencies, background-foreground confusions, auditory problems, body-concept difficulties (including space and directionality) — all of these difficulties will affect progress in reading, arithmetic, spelling, language, organization, and comprehension, as well as writing. In learning to write, many of the child's neuro-muscular functions are brought into play, thereby offering training for deficits that affect the child in all academic areas.

ADDITIONAL REFERENCES

Frostig, Marianne. *The Frostig Program for the Development of Visual Perception.* Chicago: Follett, 1964.

Gesell, Arnold, and Catherine S. Amatruda. *Developmental Diagnosis.* New York: Harper and Row, 1965.

Hellmuth, Jerome (ed.). *Learning Disorders, Vol. I.* Seattle, Wash.: Special Child Publication, 1965.

Kephart, Newell C. *The Slow Learner in the Classroom.* Columbus, Ohio: Charles E. Merrill, 1960.

Lewis, Richard A., A. A. Strauss, and L. E. Lehtinen. *The Other Child.* New York: Grune and Stratton, 1947.

A Kinesthetic Technique for Handwriting Development

Betty D. Madison

A NUMBER of children with learning difficulties also encounter writing difficulties. Some tense up at the sight of paper and pencil and frequently end up dissatisfied with their ability to remember and form written letters and numbers.

Learning to write in fingerpaint has been found helpful with some children. The very feel and ease of movement of the fingerpaint approach seems to promote a smoothness and flow in the pupil's response.

The following technique has been very useful with a number of children who encountered difficulty in remembering the patterns of symbols and/or who lacked sufficient eye-motor coordination to execute them.

The setup for fingerpainting is, of course, determined by the individual classroom situation. A sink with a formica working area is an excellent arrangement. With masking tape, mark off large rectangles. With felt pens, mark the left side of the rectangle green and the right side red. This marking helps to emphasize left-to-right progression and emphasizes the stopping point. If a work area of the above sort is not available, cookie sheets can be used quite satisfactorily.

The needs and behavior of the pupils will determine how many pupils may participate at one time.

To begin with, each pupil measures out liquid starch and pours it onto his space. He chooses one color of powdered paint with which he wants to work for that lesson period and measures it onto the liquid starch. Starch and paint can be mixed with circular strokes, going from left to right.

The instructions given the pupil will depend on his individual ability. The child who learns better kinesthetically, tactually, should close his eyes while the teacher helps him execute the pattern to be learned in the air — and then on the fingerpaint surface. There are pupils who learn faster tactually when the palm of the hand or four fingers are used rather than when just the index finger or the index and middle finger combined are used. Others do quite well with the index finger alone. The auditory learner profits from verbalization of the movement as he makes it. The visual learner may only need to be shown a model and then be able to reproduce it himself. Many times, though, a combination of more than one modality leads to faster achivement.

INSTRUCTION begins at the level of the child's needs, his way of learning, and his rate of learning. Whether he is right or left handed enters into his program planning.

The following progression was found useful for both teacher and volunteer helpers. It also allows the pupil to see and keep track of his own progress as he goes from step to step. Many times beginning strokes are taught at the same time as letter and number formation.

• Beginning strokes — straight across:

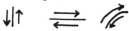

• Down - up vertical lines:

↓ ↑

• Up and down the sharp peaks:

∧∧∧∧∧∧

• Up and over the round hills:

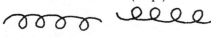

• Retrace patterns:

↓↑   ⇌   ⫽

• Ocean waves cresting to the right.

⌒⌒⌒⌒⌒⌒

• Fish on a line (loops):

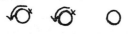

• Wriggly, squizzly snakes:

S S S S S

• Circles:

Ø Ø O

• Letters (lower case) grouped by strokes.

• Letters (lower case) combined, going from easy to more difficult combinations.

• Letters (upper case) grouped by strokes.

THE TRANSITION from fingerpaint to paper and pencil work is made whenever the pupil is ready. Most of the time, after he has mastered a stroke or letter through the media of fingerpaint, the pupil himself initiates it on paper with crayon or pencil.

With children who have difficulty making the change to paper, the following sequential steps have been useful:

• A large-lined ditto on which each stroke of the symbol is dittoed a different color. Green is used for the starting stroke and red for the stopping stroke.

• A ditto on which all strokes of the symbol are the same color.

• A ditto on which the symbol is dotted.

• A ditto on which only the starting point for the symbol is marked.

From here the child progresses to smaller-lined paper, with or without color-cued strokes or symbols as he is ready. The pupil is now on his way to successful independent writing of numbers and letters.

APPLICATION of fingerpaint techniques to the writing instruction program in this manner helps to bring about integration of kinesthetic, visual, and auditory memory for the symbol. Correct symbol formation seems to be more easily retained. Errors are quickly eliminated in fingerpaint. The pupil enjoys the experience of learning writing with this technique. Many youngsters even go back to writing in fingerpaint as their chosen "free-time" activity. This successful way of learning produces self- motivation — it's fun.

Handwriting for the Learning-Disabled

Norman Levine
Joan Carter

WITH THE IMPACT of new electronic communications equipment and supplies, handwriting might well become an obsolete skill in the next few decades. However, the ability to produce written expression satisfies some very important educational needs which no machine can supplant.

• The written word is still an important, necessary and respected form of communication. Nothing can replace the personal triumph felt by the child who writes his name for the first time.

• Beyond this, of course, the written word provides the user with a means of storing ideas and information for later retrieval.

• The ability to write affords one a means of expression and reception of language through the same skill. We can express ourselves by means of the written symbol and we can receive meaning from the written symbol, even tactually through tracing and copying.

• The written word is another avenue of expressing emotional feeling.

• The child with severely involved speech can use the written word to express his needs and feelings.

• There is status attached to the ability to write.

Letter Forms.

IN ORDER for the written material to be of use it must contain symbols that are meaningful to another, not just to the producer of the symbols. We must teach an accepted and understood form of symbols. Meaning, not perfection, then becomes the goal of the written form. Therefore, any type of letter form can be accepted as long as it can be deciphered by others. So, the form which a child uses is unimportant as long as he can shape them and communicate with them. There are three letter forms that we use.

• The first is manuscript: *and.*

• Another is cursive (generally referred to as handwriting): *and.*

• The third is a combination of both forms which can be described as *manu-cursive: and.*

Most average learners might go through the stage from manuscript to cursive rapidly but children with learning problems cling to manuscript or manu-cursive for a long time or may never leave this stage of writing.

Handwriting Sequence.

The steps to mastery in writing might be described as follows:

• There must be an awareness or recognition of the following figures: circles, half circles, triangles, squares, horizontal, vertical, and slanted lines.

• A child must have the skill to move his finger, crayon, or pencil along an indicated line.

• He must be able to follow a pencil or crayon in a groove.

• There must be the skill to follow figures and shapes presenting resistance and to trace over a figure.

• The highest skill is to copy without a pattern and reproduce figures by visual or verbal clues.

Where To Begin.

THE CHILD is asked to write his name, address, and other written words that might be familiar to him. If he is unable to do any of these, then he is asked to write or print any letter he knows. If there seems to be little skill in producing letters by his own initiative, then some commonly used letters are shown to determine if he can copy letters visually. Failing this, he is requested to draw a circle, half circle or part of a circle, vertical, horizontal, and slanted lines. If this presents a problem, then he is shown a circle and lines and again asked to produce them. Failing this, the child is asked to walk in a circle traced on the floor or marked with tape.

All of this informal testing can indicate at what level the child is able to function in handwriting skill. Handwriting moves in a certain direction

and the teacher must observe the ability of the child to move from left to right and stay on a line when writing letters. It is entirely possible for some youngsters to be able to produce certain letters easily and be unable to produce others. Sometimes a child has to be at various skill steps (as described above) to form different letters. The *b* and the *d* can be confusing to a child who has not a built-in awareness of the midline of his body and who does not know left from right. Lines which go away from the body are more easily formed than the threatening lines which come toward the body or below the lines on the paper.

Techniques.

To develop an awareness of figures, many activities can be provided. These include walking in a circle or straight line which have been marked on the surface. This same activity can be used to teach *left* and *right, backwards* and *forwards, start* and *stop, straight* and *crooked.* Adding obstacles or furniture to the area can be used to teach concepts such as *next to, in front of, sideways, toward* and *away from, between, middle,* and *before* and *after.* When the child is able to follow these directions, move from a large surface to the surface of a table top or desk.

• To teach the skill to move along a guided line, it may be necessary at first to physically guide the child's hand along the line. Place tape on the desk in the shape of a circle, lines, and half circles and allow the child to follow these with his fingers, eventually concentrating on one finger of the preferred hand. Use a chalkboard containing written figures on which the child traces with his finger and then allow him to do the same with some chalk. Using a large sheet of slick paper and allowing the child to use fingerpaint materials to produce figures adds to the enjoyment of learning. A sand table is helpful to allow the child to "feel" the figures as he makes the circles and lines.

• Permit the child to feel and identify plastic letters placed in a bag, having him give their sounds, if possible. Use many colored crayons over the same letter to reinforce the letter figure.

• The skill to move in a groove can be accomplished by using a sheet of clay with circles and lines indented. Introduce, at this point, letters such as *O, A, E,* and *F.* The use of letter templates is very good practice. The thickness of the templates should be sufficient so that the child can feel the thickness and stay within the groove. Letters cut from cardboard or felt and glued to a piece of cardboard can be used for finger tracing and used as a pattern under a sheet of paper on which a child can feel the letters.

• The skill to move with resistance can be taught by using clay also. Place the template over the clay slab and allow the child to make the letters in the clay using his finger or an orange stick. Wet sand can be used in this manner also. Letters, shapes, and forms drawn on very coarse sandpaper provide the necessary resistance effect.

• For practice in tracing over a figure, use the blackboard that has colored chalk figures on it and permit the child to use his finger over the figures and later let him use chalk. Place figures on a piece of drawing paper and let the child practice tracing these figures. Use different colors for different shapes and lines. Place a green dot to aid child in knowing where to start and a red dot to indicate the stopping point. Place shapes and lines under clear plastic and have the child trace with a grease pencil or other medium that can later be erased. Tracing paper can also be used in the same manner as described above.

• The skill to write or make a figure without a pattern is the final stage in the teaching of the handwriting sequence. At this stage, most of the above-mentioned techniques and materials can be used effectively. All that is needed are pictures of shapes, lines, and letters for the child to reproduce.

AFTER the child has the ability to reproduce shapes and lines by himself, then the letters can be presented by the above handwriting sequence, if necessary. Usually the child does not have to go back to the very first step with each letter. He may need some of the earlier techniques only if he is having difficulty with certain letters.

Little discussion has been given to the problem of writing in a relatively straight line. This can be accomplished by always providing paper with lines. It is poor procedure in writing to use unlined paper. A good type of paper to use is the heavy dark-lined paper used for children with visual impairments. Another method is to use lined paper, and block out the spaces which are to be left blank:

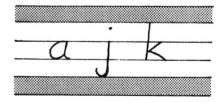

This helps the child stay in the desired space.

Following the ability to form letters, words should then be presented. The first words used should be those of importance to the writer, such as his name, address, and names of members of his family.

Each child seems to write with a different posture. It is important that each child assume the easiest posture for him. To effect this, it is helpful to tape the papers to a heavy board and allow the child to manipulate the board until he finds the most comfortable position for writing.

When the child starts to write letters and/or words, it is helpful to have him verbalize these letters and words as he writes. This can be of inestimable help in developing sound-symbol relationships which will prove useful in reading.

Remember to allow the child to use whatever letter form is easiest for him. If a transition is desired, it can always be introduced at a later time.

Begin instruction at the level at which the child is functioning. It provides the success needed by the learning disabled child.

The Vulnerable Child and Cursive Writing

Norma Banas

I. H. Wills

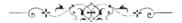

WE ARE ALL equipped with sensors which are stimulated by all parts of our environment. In order to sort this mass of stimulation, we are also equipped with dampening devices, a control panel, and a monitoring system.

The Vulnerable Child is equally equipped with sensors, but his dampeners may be malfunctioning or the selective controls are less discrete. Instead of a smooth band or continuum from total awareness to subconscious awareness, the sensors seem either to be attending to everything or tuning out completely.

The one thing the Vulnerable Child seems unable to do is to stay tuned in for any length of time to selected stimuli. If he turns his attention from any immediate stimuli, he has a great deal of trouble in regaining the same tuning. Hence, he may learn something well on one occasion; but, unless an identical situation occurs, he does not recognize the common element in the two experiences and cannot use what he learned. In some instances, he may have a distorted perception because he is reacting in totality — reacting to the differences as well as to the common elements. Thus, he has perceptual confusion and his learning pattern is uneven.

One of the major complaints of teachers is the poor cursive formation of the Vulnerable Child. The key to writing and reading in cursive is the establishment of association between the printed and the cursive word. Through a step-by-step kinesthetic-associative approach, the child can conceptualize and visualize the cursive process as the printed form which has been connected. By the addition of a meaningful picture clue to the usual tracing step for recall reinforcement, the child has a concrete association of a specific idea. This is especially important for the nontangible words in our language — the very words that seem to be most difficult for the Vulnerable Child to hold.

Kina-writing is an associative approach to cursive writing which has been found to be an important technique used in heightening the visualization of words to aid recall of sight vocabulary, spelling, or meaning vocabulary, and with phonics skills development. It must be taught carefully so that problems of figure-ground, directionality, or spatial organization, and the problems created by printing taught as a segmented process can be eliminated. Once this technique is established as a successful activity, it can be used by children independently for reinforcement of vocabulary or spelling at all levels, in any context, and with foreign languages.

PRESCRIPTIVE TEACHING GUIDE
(Kina-writing – for third grade and up.)
Materials: Strips of white tagboard, 4½″ x 11″(kina-cards).
Procedure: Take words from any book in which the child is working and which may need recall reinforcement and direct the child through the following steps:

• COPY each word, one word to a kina-card, in pencil. Proper and exaggerated spatial relations are needed to fully involve the child kinesthetically and to heighten his perception of the word configuration. (Copy about five words per lesson.) Check for accuracy of copy and letter formation.

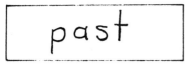

• DRAW A PICTURE on the back of each card to illustrate the meaning of the word. Teacher or parent must check, at first, for correctness and accuracy of meaning. Thinking *who, what, when, where, why, how* helps the student make his pictogram fully meaningful.

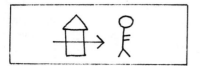

• CONNECT each letter, using the crayon, so the finished work appears in cursive form. (At first, teacher illustrates on the board using two chalk colors.) Careful guidance is needed at this step where directionality and eye-hand coordination problems may interfere with the child's execution of this stage. (Check before tracing.)

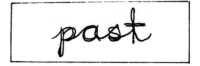

• TRACE a word three times with the crayon *as* the student says the word quietly but aloud. (Be sure the student keeps his arm from resting on the table. Freedom of movement as well as large movements are important. Write the word on the chalkboard with eyes closed. Check the model. Retrace if incorrect. Do each word in turn.

• FILE words in a shoe box, in *ABC* order, for use as flashcards.

The following instructions are suggested when introducing the connective step:

Swing up to where the letter begins when you print . . . make your letter as always, swing up to the next letter, make an . . ., etc.

Note that it is often necessary to correct the child's directionality by placing an arrow to remind him that all letters move from left to right as they are formed, and that we begin at the top of each letter. Segmenting manuscript letters is detrimental to the child with directional or eye-hand coordination problems.

Always teach with words, never as letters in isolation. For some children it will be necessary to print the word for him until he has sufficient eye-hand control. For those with a figure-ground problem, color used for the printed word helps him to be able to follow when he connects and traces.

At first, avoid words containing an *r*, *s*, *f*, or *z*. These are the only let-

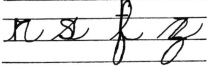

ters which change from the printed form.

The technique described above provides a means by which the Vulnerable Child can make a relatively smooth transition from the printed to the cursive letter form. The devices of the pictogram and the use of color are designed to fix the visual image of the word in the child's mind so that he can recognize it when he sees it in other situations. It is through careful reinforcement such as this that the Vulnerable Child will be aided in reaching his full achievement capacity.

a b c d e f g h i j k

l m n o p q r s t u

v w x y z

Outlining was a new
thing for me
seperating ideas from
details we see
facts in the
enciclopedia I never
saw before
E.D.S. Made outlining
important and
not a bore
by Bob
8th grade

Solving Early Reading Problems Via Handwriting

E. A. Enstrom and Doris C. Enstrom

———————————•••————————————

THERE IS NO DENYING that we have a multitude of learning problems in the early school years. Dr. Kiyoshi Makita, director of the Children's Psychiatric Service, Keio University School of Medicine, Tokyo, calls attention to the 15 percent of all pupils in America who have reading problems compared to fewer than 1 percent of Japanese children. Nor should we overlook that in Japan reading is infinitely more difficult because of the ideographs plus forty-eight symbols that stand for sound. Therefore, to teach children to learn to read Japanese requires real instructional effort which is accompanied by learning to write the symbols.[1]

Also, we note that in the i/t/a program, which is a writing approach to reading, the forty-four symbols have to be initially learned during the first two months of school — a task requiring genuine teaching effort. Here it is reported that there is a reduction in general learning disability, including the so-called "perception" problems.

Makita gives credit for the lack of problems to the language system itself. Is this the correct answer, or is the intensive early instructional effort to learn to write the symbols the reason for lack of failure?

For over three decades in America, using the traditional approaches, instead of exerting herculean efforts in mastery of a language system, teachers have been encouraged to deemphasize the importance of handwriting and have been encouraged to produce an easy-going environment of play, without exact requirements being prescribed. Children have been asked to write meaningful material before they have learned to write. Mistakes, wrong moves, incorrect sequence, etc., have been shrugged off as unimportant while incidental approaches have been encouraged. As a result, many early handwriting problems have been permitted to become established as habit. This, I contend, is responsible for many of our serious reading problems from which fifteen percent of our children suffer.

Reports show that children with learning disability, in addition to having reading problems, *always* reverse letters, invert letters, place letters and numerals

[1] News Front, *Phi Delta Kappan*, 50 (November 1968), p. 198.

on the side, mirror their writing, and in general have numerous handwriting problems. These errors have been reported as *additional* problems. From our observation over many years in working with all types of disability, such writing *is the cause* of reading problems. Such errors are not just a tag-along relationship.

While others have eliminated or prevented most problems by having children master a very difficult language situation which involves both handwriting and reading, in many schools of this country the trend has been toward slighting the mastery of a well organized handwriting program and emphasizing reading alone. We would suggest that many problems could be solved by greater emphasis on early handwriting instruction, properly programmed.

Why are there so many problems?

In America, because of an abundance of newspapers, magazines, books, T.V. programs, etc., in the average home, children often try to write during very early years. These children are usually bright and have a strong desire to do as their elders are doing. In secret, or for all the world to see, they copy material from seemingly unlimited environmental sources.

Problems are born because these early efforts are, too often, unguided. No one tells the child where to begin, which direction to move, which sequence of parts to follow. No one tells him which hand to use or how to hold the pencil. Often, when writing from memory, he reverses letters, lays them on the side, or even places them completely upside down. Every time he repeats the error, he is fixing the habit more firmly. Upon arrival at school, these wrong moves tend to persist. The incidental approach advocated by many past educators tends to encourage teachers to overlook these early wrong moves and shrug them off with the thought, "Oh, well, he will soon grow out of it."

But the sad fact is, the child *does not* grow out of it, and the reason he does not is because of this psychological fact: All early efforts, whether right or wrong, tend to be repeated and become firmly established as habit.

When the incorrect process finally begins to interfere with progress in reading, teachers begin pushing the panic button, calling for psychological help, and thus begins the process of figuring out a new name with a true professional ring that adequately described the reason for the failure. There is a tendency to become so enthralled by the name that the child and his problem are often lost in the shuffle.[2]

Too often, the average classroom teacher, for fear of further damaging the child, is reluctant to apply the long overdue teaching. The problem and, indeed, the disability get increasingly serious with each passing year of frustration for the child.

Let us begin by teaching children how to hand write.

In rooms where much emphasis is placed upon correct early learning of handwriting, these problems tend not to exist or are few and minimized. When

---

[2]Edward Fry contributes to the naming game with "Do-It-Yourself Terminology Generator," *Journal of Reading*, 11 (March 1968), 428. This is recommended reading for everyone.

letters are placed in all directions in handwriting, there can possibly be nothing but reading problems. Reading and handwriting are strongly intertwined.[3] A well planned handwriting program can prevent many potential problems *before they become problems.*

Reversals, inversions, etc., can usually be overcome by proceeding in the following manner:

Begin by teaching the basic left-to-right direction, as in Figure 1. Place much emphasis on *listening* and *watching.* Place equal emphasis on *pupils' learning to follow directions.*

Figure 1

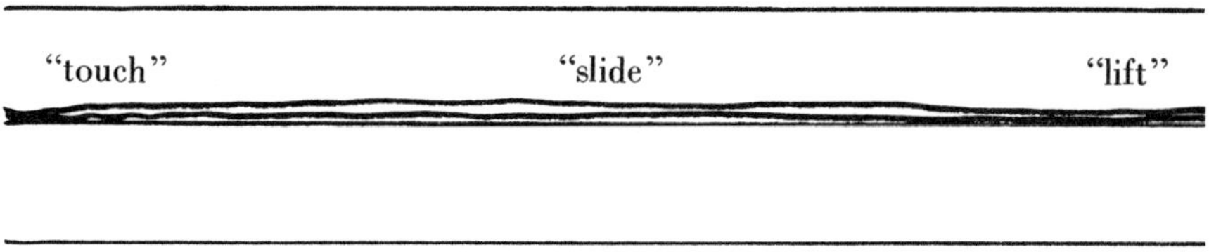

"touch"   "slide"   "lift"

Move left to right only while using this initial print writing exercise. Have pupils say aloud, "touch, slide, lift," "touch, slide, lift," and repeat it many times. *Establish this as habit.*

Next, practice the same direction in short, *untraced* strokes that so often appear in print letters and numerals. This is seen in Figure 2.

Figure 2

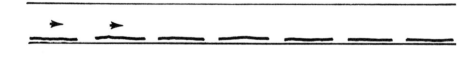

Again, have children say aloud, "touch, slide," "touch, slide," while practicing. Do not leave these exercises until all children *habitually* move in the left-to-right direction.[4]

Many times when a child writes at a high desk, he begins at the point closest to his body and moves upward for vertical strokes. The next *habit*, then, to be established is the necessity of moving from the top downward at all times.

[3]Evelyn Mae White, "Teaching 'Discovery-Linguistics,' " *Elementary English,* 45 (March 1968), 342-345.

[4]Used with the permission of Peterson Handwriting, Greensburg, Pennsylvania.

The right length can be established by "building a fence" with the long-line exercises. Skip one line as in Figure 3. Then begin at the top and make *untraced* down strokes two spaces long. Usually this "fence" is sufficient to obtain the desired length of strokes. In extreme cases, one can use a strip of masking tape at the top and another two spaces down. Keep the downstrokes between the two pieces of tape. But as with all crutches, get rid of these guides as soon as possible. Independent work is the goal. Incidentally, tape guides are also valuable at the chalkboard. They can be used to obtain vertical strokes as well as to indicate stops.

Figure 3

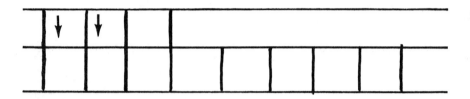

Next, practice downward strokes one space high. It is very important in all cases to have the children say *aloud* what they are doing: "Touch, down," "touch, down," etc.

From these basic habits it is easy to build letters with *no reversals, inversions, or on-the-side placements,* as in Figure 4.

Figure 4

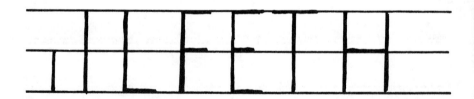

Because of previously learned incorrect habits, children must be watched lest they lapse into former ways. Seat problem cases near the center front where they can be easily watched and helped while the teacher is working with the group. Chalkboard writing is another solution to the watching problem, but with careful, exacting teaching, problems of deviation from instruction are rare, indeed.

If there are serious deviations, review often, always saying aloud what is to be done. Occasional individualized instruction will usually eliminate any wrong moves. In extreme cases where a child has been permitted to establish a multitude of wrong directional moves, the transfer to paper can be simplified by (a) learning to write correctly on the chalkboard, (b) practicing on large paper fastened to the chalkboard with tape, (c) then taking the paper to the desk and continuing writing the "over and down" exercises or letters.

The next teaching task should be the development of the rounded (but not round) family of letters. If one begins with an "umbrella" touching the top line, he can easily establish the all-important correct beginning point and direction of motion.

In making "umbrellas," begin at the right and move *leftward* as in Figure 5.

Figure 5

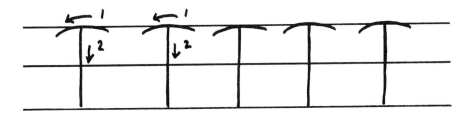

Beginning point and direction of the top are very important in order to prevent incorrect movement for this often used group of letters. Children usually have a good mental picture of an umbrella, and this exercise establishes both the round top for the C-family and the correct direction of motion.

Incidentally, problems are solved or reduced by having pupils *always* encircle items in workbooks in this counter-clockwise direction.

Next, continue the "umbrella" top on around for making capital C and eventually add the cross bar for making G as in Figure 6. There is no educational merit in making G a complex, difficult letter.

Figure 6

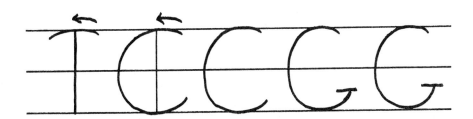

Repeat these two letters many times to establish as habit the very important beginning point and direction of motion. If there is much difficulty in touching lines have pupils say aloud, "touch" as they near the top line and "touch" as they approach the base line. This is very helpful in obtaining greater accuracy with the rounded group.

From the well established *C*, reduce the size to one space and gradually teach the "seven *c*'s" family as seen in Figure 7.

Figure 7

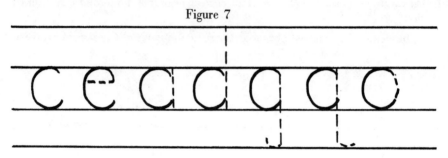

Because of both "similarity and difference" there will always be reversal confusion with lower case *d* and *b*. It is the *d* that causes most problems, but this can be controlled by having children say *aloud* while practicing *d*'s, "*c* comes before *d*," "*c* comes before *d*." While saying this aloud, children make the *c*, then add the long line to make it a *d*, as in Figure 8.

Figure 8

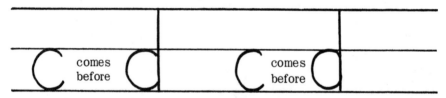

Reversals with capital *S* are eliminated by alternations capitals *C* and *S* – "they begin the same way." If necessary, bring in more "umbrellas" as in Figure 9. Next, reduce the size and alternate small *c* and *s*.

Figure 9

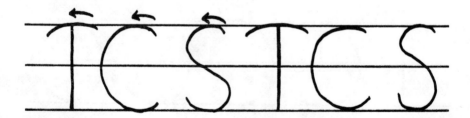

The *N* reversal is solved by very exacting instruction. Have children practice stroke-by-stroke under the teacher's direction. Make the two upright (vertical) lines. Then have everybody place his pencil at the top of the first one and keep it there until all pencils are so placed. Only then direct the children to move to the bottom of the second line. Repeat several times and thus establish the correct learning.

Formal teaching.

We hear criticism such as: "But all this sounds so formal and children are really not writing any meaningful things." We have our choice — either teach initial handwriting stroke-by-stroke under the exact directions of the teacher — controlled all the way, or continue having reversals, mirroring, and inversions along with our high fifteen percent learning disability problems! It is a choice instructors must make.

Early formal instruction is no worry to us — we have taught and directed the teaching of thousands of children — including classes labeled "perception" as well as many other problem groups. Either no problems evolved or former problems vanished by using the above approaches. One point is significant for teachers: There is nothing quite so important as "right the first time." Educators are finally awakening to the fact that it is much easier and less wasteful to prevent problems in the first place than it is to "cure" them later. And most of our problems are the "cure-them-later" variety. Early, exacting instruction would have prevented most of them from ever happening.

Once all letters have been correctly learned with proper placement — there will be time for wide informal use of the correct writing tool. Indeed, after each group of letters has been learned, more and more meaningful words, phrases, and short sentences can be practiced. At the beginning we need to be more concerned with correct, "no-problem" writing than with using a half-learned tool that later causes confusion with all related areas, including spelling and reading.

Two new developments help the teacher in the very important stroke-by-stroke correct learning: (a) The Colorgraph presentation of letter shapes. Here adequate attention has been given to direction and sequence. Incidentally, this developmental technique is now available on transparencies for the overhead projector.[5] By flashing these *on the chalkboard* the instructor can easily individualize the teaching. Simply have pupils trace the steps, erase, then trace again. (b) The second new development is the wider use of the overhead projector in teaching handwriting. For initial instruction this device is especially important because on the screen the image is like a moving picture. The child sees an enlarged picture of the teacher's pencil and hand as it touches the correct spot; at the same time the hand and pencil shadow reveals the direction of movement as well as the part which follows. This enlarged presentation is superior to a chalkboard presentation. Teachers are urged to make wide use of the tools available for improved instruction, which, without question, reduces the mountain of unnecessary problems.

W E WOULD SUGGEST THAT many of our so-called "perception" and other problems have their source — or at least are associated with — early untutored writing habits established in the home. Nor can we forget the trend in

---

[5]Projectuals for Print Colorgraph; Projectuals for Cursive Colorgraph. Greensburg, Pa.: Peterson Handwriting. New York: The Macmillan Company.

some American schools to neglect careful instruction in handwriting. We are reaping the "rewards" of incidental instruction and the foolishness of trying to use a skill before correct ways have been adequately mastered. Having tried everything else, now let us try *success through careful initial teaching of handwriting.*

The sooner we abandon the "do-it-in-the-most-comfortable-way" philosophy and emphasize instead, "right-the-first-time," the sooner success will emerge. The more care that is taken with instructing initial correct ways in handwriting, the earlier we shall arrive at an elimination of most reading problems.

Stress Reduction and Handwriting

Harris L. PreFontaine

WHEN I WENT to grade school it was customary that the desks be placed so that the windows were on the left of the child. Bright days forced all heads to be tipped to the left in order to block out the glare. Seldom were lights turned on except on particularly dark days and then, of course, there was the problem of seeing around the shadow caused by the ineffective lighting.

We were taught, as effectively as our environment would allow, a system of penmanship called "Palmer Method." As I recall, the posture instructions were, "Sit alert with back slightly away from the chair back, pencil held about an inch from the point so that the point can be seen with both eyes, and with arms on the desk in a comfortable position," etc.

In my opinion, the practice of assuming the recommended posture did, in fact, counteract the disadvantages of the lighting and glare in our environment. The end result was better penmanship, as well as better visual and body posture — in spite of the architecture and lighting. When practicing the "Palmer Method" posture we, no doubt, corrected some of the body postures induced into the posture behavior patterns by the light-

ing and the flat desks or tables (which are still used in some schools).

Today, through the influence of such people as Darell Boyd Harmon, Gesell, and many others, the new architecture has eliminated many of the old problems. Training of the proper posture for hand-eye coordination also seems to have been eliminated from many school systems.

Because there are no shadows or glare to contend with in the modern classroom, it would seem that many teachers find it less necessary to instruct the child in the proper method of holding a pencil or pen and in proper posture. I would like teachers to really look at the postures of the children in the classroom as they are attempting to write.

SO MANY children who are brought in for a visual case study because they do not seem to be achieving up to their intellectual potential have poor handwriting, and they show, on testing, a so-called "neuro-confusion factor." This "neuro-confusion" has, in fact, been described as dyslexia.

Observing the writing posture of these children, it is noted that their method of holding the pencil has

35

forced their head to the left (if right handed) in order to guide the point of the pencil with at least one eye. This, in turn, forces a suppression of the other eye, thereby increasing the effectiveness of the opposite eye from the handedness.

G. N. Getman states:

Children must learn to use and control themselves before they learn to use and control elaborate equipment. In fact, the child always possessed his own learning equipment, and it is the control and use of the equipment that establishes the basis for all other learning.[1]

The improperly learned behavior can in some measure be responsible for retarding the child's intellectual development. Eye-hand relationships have been shown to be a part of the perceptual development of the child.

IN THE OPINION of many optometrists working with nonachieving children, many things can be done in the schools preventatively. Prevention of any problem is usually easier than its correction and this may be true of slow-learning children. For example:

• Use tilt-top tables and desks for crayon and pencil activities.

• Give proper instruction for holding the pencil or crayon so that both eyes can guide the point.

• Give instruction in the proper body positioning for writing and reading.

These few basic suggestions, if consistently followed, particularly from kindergarten through grade three,

could lead to better eye-hand relationships, thus preventing some neuroconfusion and slow-learning factors.

Many of the problems of the slow-learning child seem to be aggravated by over-stress which apparently is induced by the lack of proper behavioral patterns.

"We grow toward over-stress to reduce stress." Darell Boyd Harmon has dramatically demonstrated this fact both in movies and in his book, *The Coordinated Classroom.*[2]

He states:

The work environment of the immature organism (the child) must be equally coordinated with the organ itself if we would have the child arrive at an optimum maturity, fully capable of using its resources and developmental experiences in meeting its needs in an efficient, acceptable, and satisfying manner. (p. 1)

According to C. Judson Herrick:[3]

Although the energy expended in mental effort is quantitatively small, intelligence is the most precious acquisition on our planet and when efficiently and judiciously used it yields the largest profit. As we shall see, the specific properties of mind are better described in terms of patterns of performance and patterns of relations rather than quantitatively in terms of energy or anything else. This has long been recognized by some and is now accepted by our most competent authorities.

In the examination of mind we are looking not at a particu-

---

[1]G. N. Getman, "Optometric Child Care and Guidance," *Optometric Extension Papers*, XXXIII (May 1961).

[2](Grand Rapids, Michigan: American Seating Co., 1949.)

[3]*The Evolution of Human Nature* (Austin, Texas: University of Texas Press, 1956).

lar kind of thing but at a distinctive kind of process. What we observe is a *minding body*, not a body that makes a separate entity called the mind . . . When we observe a thinking man we must not separate the action from the actor. A vital process, we repeat, cannot split apart in this way. (pp. 288-289)

Overt behavior is movement of some sort. Movement is primordial and mentation arises within it not to cause behavior but to regulate it, direct it, and improve its efficiency. Conscious emotive experience reinforces the action system with additional driving power, and in proportion as intelligence guides the direction taken in its expression, the efficiency of the behavior is improved. (p. 312)

It is only as the body reacts to the retinal image by directive (purpose-like) movement that the sensory stimuli acquire significance. (p. 348)

Montessori, who speaks of "the pedagogical method of observation," says that "the education of the senses makes men observers." Such education has as its aim "the refinement of the differential perception of stimuli by means of repeated exercises . . . The degree of success of the teacher will be largely determined by her ability as an observer."[4]

THE POSTURES and habits developed in early elementary grades are very difficult to reverse later. Perhaps we should take a closer look at the children while they are learning to color and write in kindergarten through the third grade. Perhaps we should also take a closer look at what the flat-top work tables are doing to the hand-eye relationships and body postures of these young children.

Perhaps we should then reevaluate what these faulty behavior patterns do to learning ability and comprehension in higher grades.

_____

[4]R. C. Orem (ed.), *A Montessori Handbook* (New York: G. P. Putnam's Sons, 1965).

I didn't like school-I was on the
wrong path.
I thought I was a fool because
I didn't like math.
But then I saw light.
Everything seemed bright.
Egs cleared away the bad day.
And then I was gay.

by Nancy
4th grade

Remedial Approaches
to Handwriting Dysfunction

Shirley Linn

TO WRITE, a person must produce meaningful symbols on paper which communicate thoughts to others. This must occur in a manner which has meaning to both sender and receiver. Children with learning disabilities or a neurological impairment often have problems that interfere with the production of symbols which will communicate thoughts meaningfully.

Specific problems experienced by these children are: poor construction of letters, such as lines which cross instead of meeting or which meet instead of crossing; corners which turn at irregular angles; lines which gape; poor or irregular letter size (some tall, some short, regardless of the size they should be); difficulty with letters which go above the line, below the line, and those which do both; reversals; inversions; poor spacing; poor placement or position on lines or between lines and spaces.

These errors are symptomatic of developmental lags or deficiency which may occur singly or in combination. They are usually associated with problems in such areas as motor development, language development (receptive, associative, or expressive), or visual perception. Writing itself is con-

sidered a motor skill, but it is one which is dependent on the ability of the individual to integrate separate skills into expressive action.

Traditionally, children are given lessons for handwriting which include oral directions by the teacher, illustrations on the chalkboard, writing in the air, and then application on paper at a desk. This approach assumes the child is capable of understanding directions which are given orally, illustrations which are given visually, and that he is also able to interpret and carry out the directions given. Carrying out directions is dependent on motor ability, the ability to perceive the space in which one lives and the space on which one writes, as well as the ability to translate oral directions into expressive action.

A child with learning disabilities is often unable to establish a keen understanding of directionality, laterality, or a concept of himself in his physical environment. Most children learn about their position in space through the movements of their body when they move, turn, crawl, pull up, walk, run, etc. In every action, they should learn more about themselves in terms of space and their relationship to it. Children with developmental lag need assistance to learn to control and coordinate gross motor muscles. Remediation at this stage should include many experiences with their environment. For more complete assessment of the role of motor development and remediation, the reader is referred to the works of other authors.[1]

THE PROBLEMS of a student with an unstable understanding of himself in his environment are compounded when he is given directions for writing lessons. His understanding of directions for space-related activities is often limited. The words *up, down, slant, slide,* up until the time when he is told to sit at a desk and write, indicate directions in space oriented to his upright position. Once he sits at the desk, the words take on new meaning. The point of reference changes from the upright position to the horizontal plane on the desk. Children with learning disabilities, insecure in their own positions in space, are unable to make the transfer or to understand the change in reference. Therefore, their ability to comprehend the directions may be deficient.

Remediation includes exercises which enable a child to learn to listen, comprehend, then follow directions. They include orientation of the child toward understanding of names

for places and positions in his environment in relation to his own position. Direct application of vocabulary to teach changes from upright to horizontal may be made by utilizing a hard surface such as a tablet on a clipboard, which can be brought from the upright to the horizontal position gradually as lessons are taught. This, according to Frostig, enables a youngster to make the necessary transfer of vocabulary and its application from one position to another.[2]

ONCE control is gained in gross motor development, it should progress to finer muscles. Just as these children needed more structured activities to develop control over large muscles, they need structured activities to develop control over fine muscles. They need more than the usual amount of experience with play activities, such as playing with blocks, simple puzzles, cars, dolls, and other typical preschool play activities. These activities assist in development of control over finer muscles.

Children who have difficulty with ordinary play activity receive little pleasure from it and tend to avoid it. This gives them even less opportunity to develop the skills that play activities promote. For children who do not learn to play naturally, it is often necessary to teach them as one would teach an academic activity. This involves study of the skills needed and a step-by-step presentation of the activity, being sure that each step is mastered before going on to the next. Once mastered the activity is more enjoyable, is used more often, and in turn provides the needed practice.

[1]Newell C. Kephart, *The Slow Learner in the Classroom* (Columbus, Ohio: Charles E. Merrill, 1961); D. H. Radler and N. C. Kephart, *Success Through Play* (New York: Harper and Brothers, 1960); Eugene G. Roach and N. C. Kephart, *The Purdue Perceptual Motor Survey* (Columbus, Ohio: Charles E. Merrill, 1966); Marianne Frostig and David Horne, *The Frostig Program for Development of Visual Perception* (Chicago, Ill.: Follett, 1964).

[2]*Ibid.*, p. 20.

As skill in preschool play activities improves, scribbling activities usually follow. As children master scribbling, they learn to match the visual trace with the lines made. They learn to produce lines, associate them with directions on paper, and to make the hands work independently of the eyes and the eyes work independently of the hands.

More structured activities often are necessary prior to the time writing can actually be taught. Children with lags in development need structured activities such as those provided by the Frostig Program for Development of Visual Perception. Especially helpful are the visual-motor coordination series. Children need to learn to listen to instructions which tell them to make lines in specific directions. These activities include verbal instructions which assist this development. As the child progresses through the worksheets, all important direction words are taught. Some children need even more emphasis on directions and their meaning. They need understanding of directions which relate to them personally. Directions such as, "Touch the bottom of the plate — the side closest to you," help children orient themselves to the space they are in and the space on which they are writing. Frequent review of directions, as the child sees them from his own focal point, is essential.

Difficulty in understanding directions and carrying them out is closely interwoven with the problems of motor coordination and visual perception. For example, children having difficulty seeing and making lines cross will receive help from visual-perceptual training in the areas of figure-ground. Also helpful is a good writing system which uses color cues. Children who make letters of all sorts of sizes and all over each space will benefit from exercises in sections relating to spatial relations, position in space, and perceptual constancy.[3]

IT IS IMPORTANT to give a great deal of thought to the writing system used. Many good systems are available today, but those which use color seem most effective. These cues seem to provide the stimulus to remain in the general vicinity of the appropriate place to write. They help children see when lines cross, intersect, and turn. One very good system is the *Peterson Directed Handwriting Series,* which uses color cues skillfully.[4] This series uses color to designate the area to be used for writing, black lines going across the page from left to right to show where letters are to be placed, colored lines showing directional differences, and directional arrows to show the way to make the strokes for letters. In addition, proper sequence of line construction is shown by giving the strokes numbers.

For some children, however, the color cues may be inadequate. Raised letters are sometimes needed for reinforcement through touching or tracing. This is often helpful with beginners as well as with children with persistent problems. Cards can be made to show how lines cross to form letters. First, letters are traced on cards with pencil. A thin line of glue is then used to trace the line, and yarn is placed on the glue. Variegated yarn can best provide the variety of color needed to coordinate colors of cards with the writing system used. When possible, children should make their own cards. In this way they can learn to see how lines cross, turn, change directions in order to become meaningful symbols. Once complete

---

[3]Frostig, *op. cit.*
[4](New York: Macmillan, 1968.)

the cards can be used again and again for tracing. It is important to reduce the tactile structure as soon as possible so it will not become a crutch. Tactile surfaces can be reduced by using only glue to outline the letters.

The system described above can assist children to see that different parts are used to make letters. Letters themselves should be combined to make words as soon as possible in order for the children to see that letters are parts of words and that they represent sounds.

TO SUMMARIZE, the ability to communicate with written symbols on paper is often a determining factor in whether a youngster is able to achieve academically or not. Children with otherwise normal ability are often unable to put their thoughts on paper, not because of thinking disorders, but rather because of writing disorders.

Until recently, writing disorders were considered primarily motor problems. With more study of motor and perceptual development, it has become evident that developmental lag can affect writing ability. Using this approach, it is possible to reach and work at the source of the problem, thereby reducing the incidence of a writing disability that becomes a permanent affliction rather than a temporary symptom.

ADDITIONAL REFERENCES

Gesell, Arnold, and Catherine Amatruda. *Developmental Diagnosis.* New York: Harper and Brothers, 1948.

Gesell, Arnold, and Frances C. Ilg. *The Child From Five to Ten.* New York: Harper and Brothers, 1946.

Kindergarten Practices, 1961. Research Monograph, 1962-M2. Washington, D.C.: Research Division, National Education Assn., 1962.

Sears, Pauline, and Edith M. Dowley. "Research on Teaching in the Nursery School," *Handbook of Research on Teaching.* Edited by N. L. Gage. Chicago: Rand McNally, 1963.

Standing, E. M. *The Montessori Method.* Fresno, Calif.: Academy Library Guild, 1962.

Handwriting and Correct Posture

Ben Croutch

———— ✠ ————

BASIC difficulties in handwriting often center around posture. It is possible to help the greater percentage of youngsters having handwriting trouble by having them adjust to a correct writing posture. I refer here to students whose writing is illegible or who have difficulty writing at a normal speed.[1]

A left-handed person, in many cases, is accepted as a poor writer when in reality a few minor corrections could help to improve his or her writing. Most left handers have been permitted to turn the paper the same way as for a right-handed individual. In some cases, the teacher walking down the aisle of a class has caused the child to turn the paper the wrong way in order that the teacher may read his paper. After the teacher has returned to her desk, the child's paper remains in the same position.

The position of the paper for a left-handed writer should be with the bottom right-hand corner pointing at the child's navel. Thus, if you drew or extended a line from the navel to the right-hand corner and continued in a straight line, it would bisect the paper at the upper left-hand corner.

A right-handed writer would have the paper turned so that the bottom left-hand corner would be pointing at the navel. This simple positioning of the paper, in many cases, will alleviate a basic problem of the poor writer. It is important that this correct position of paper be stressed; one cannot gradually move the paper to the correct position, trying to overcome a child's bad habit.

The right hand of the left-handed writer should be resting on the bottom half of the paper with the lower arm off the desk. The reverse is true for the right-handed writer. This position will allow the writer a more extensive visual field when writing. The body also will be in better balance, thus putting less strain on the entire body, including the eyes, and providing for a relaxed writing posture.

The elbow and forearm of the writing hand must be on the desk. This provides for freedom of movement when writing. As you can see, if the

---

[1] This article is not designed to catalog the reasons for a handicap in handwriting. See Anna Gillingham and Bessie Stillman, *Remedial Training for Children with Specific Disability in Reading, Spelling, and Penmanship* (Cambridge, Mass.: Educators Publishing Service, 1960); Darrell Boyd Harmon, "A Preliminary Report on a Study of Eye Preference, Certain Body Mechanics, and Visual Problems," *Learning Disorders, II* ed. Jerome Hellmuth (Seattle: Special Child Publications, 1965).

elbow of the writing hand is always to be on the desk, the paper must be moved. If, instead of moving the elbow of the writing arm up and down, the paper is moved, it would prevent the wrist from turning up, thus preventing a basic problem in the poor writer. It would help also to keep the entire body in balance and alignment.

The body should be torqued (turned) to the left for the right-handed writer and to the right for a left-handed person. The back should be humped slightly (kyphosis position). The distance from the eyes to the paper should be approximately sixteen inches. This distance, for a balanced and stress-free position, is when the mid-point between the eyes, the elbow, and the knuckle of the middle finger roughly describes a right triangle, with the elbow bent approximately ninety degrees.

Furniture for the youngster is quite important to good handwriting. For the most efficient writing, with regard to eye alignment, the desk should be sloped at a twenty - degree angle. The chair and desk should be at a height that, when the student is seated with his feet flat on the floor, if his forearms are extended, they would rest in a position on the desk parallel to the floor.

THE PRECEDING information, it is hoped, will be of benefit to the poor handwriter, but one must remember that working with the youngster who has a specific writing disability may be a slow, painstaking process.

To review, the correct body alignment for writing is as follows:

• Position of paper: lower corner of paper pointing to the navel. For the right-handed writer this would be the left corner; for the left-handed writer it would be the right corner.

• Non-writing hand: resting on the lower half of the paper with forearm off the desk.

• Writing hand: forearm and elbow must be on the desk.

• Body position: turned to the left for the right-handed writer and to the right for the left-handed writer. Kyphosis position of the back.

• Eyes: sixteen inches from the paper.

Correct body posture in writing can help to prevent eye defects that may occur later in the student.

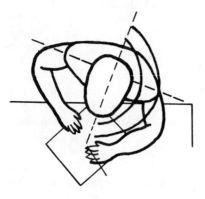
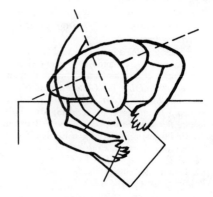

A Musical Approach to Handwriting

Ruth Iogha
Lotte Kaliski

A MUSICAL APPROACH to handwriting is an idea which evolved after working with a particular little girl who was having difficulty with visuomotor tasks, particularly handwriting, at the Kaliski School. One of the greatest strengths of this child was in the auditory area, especially in music and rhythm. It was because of these special strengths, combined with her needs, that the approach to be described was created. Although the same idea was used with several other children, the results were particularly interesting and successful with the child about whom this paper is written.

Joan came to the Kaliski School at the age of seven. This neatly groomed, friendly, and cooperative little girl, with twinkling dark eyes and tiny stature, was never at a loss for words. She sought and immediately received the attention of those around her, bringing forth their smiles and laughter.

Joan's friendly disposition enabled her to get along well with other children and she has continued to show more initiative and self-assurance each year. She became better organized, although if she can get someone to "do it for her," she will. Verbalization was her strength and one got a much better picture of her abilities through her oral contributions than through her written expressions.

From background information given us by her mother, we learned that although Joan was a full-term baby and birth was normal, she weighed only five pounds, four ounces. She assumed a standing position while holding on to supports at five months; sat alone at nine months; and stood alone at a year and a half. She did not walk until she was two years old; however, "Once she walked, she walked. No trial and error!" Her first word was spoken before she was a year old, but quite a while passed before sentences, even phrases, evolved. Physical coordination of large muscles in executing skips, gallops, balancing on roller and ice skates, riding a tricycle developed by the age of four, although these skills were never perfected to a degree equal to that of other children. Small muscle movements were conspicuously slower and at the time Joan entered the Kaliski School, she was still finding it difficult to tie shoes, button her coat, cut, draw, put together puzzles, write, etc.

At first, it was felt that Joan was a slow developer, and she repeated kindergarten to give the maturational processes more time. Medical tests, however, diagnosed Joan as being minimally brain damaged. Placement in a special school for children with learning disabilities was suggested.

PRIOR TO admission to the Kaliski School, we received several reports pertaining to Joan's level of functioning in various areas. On a psychometric evaluation several years ago, Joan was seen as perseverative, easily distracted, and with a short attention span. She was quite talkative, sometimes inappropriately. On subtests involving comprehension and language usage, Joan scored above her chronological age level. Qualitatively speaking, her greatest gain had been in verbalization and vocabulary development. Items on subtests involving abstraction showed a scoring below her age level. Handedness was not at that time stabilized and she transferred the pencil from one hand to the other. A Stanford-Binet Intelligence Test (L-M) placed Joan in the dull-normal range.

Another evaluation at a later date again verified the marked visuo-motor difficulties. She was unable to draw a human figure although she could designate all parts on her own body. Joan attempted to write her name but she had the greatest difficulty in forming single letters. She omitted curves on letters and showed reversal tendencies. Right-handedness had, by this time, been established. Her auditory recall for meaningful material was fairly good. Verbalization again showed growth and remained her greatest strength.

AS PART of her program of training at the Kaliski School, Joan participated in sessions of perceptual motor training, spatial orientation, in order to help her develop a better awareness of space and to increase her coordination of both large and small muscle movements. She improved in balance, walking forward and sidewise, but had difficulty projecting space behind her when walking backwards. Difficulties in eye-hand and eye-foot coordination were apparent. Joan was not completely aware of the accurate location of her body parts or of her limits in space at any one time. Continued practice at tasks designed to develop better judgment of space between her body and external objects was beneficial. Perception of forms improved, although Joan had, at first, motor difficulty in reproducing forms. She was eager to do puzzles but needed help in manipulating the pieces.

Drawings were mostly scribbling, sometimes circular and zigzag. Body image drawings were incomplete. She worked very slowly at these tasks, needing a great deal of coaxing and reassuring before becoming involved. Painting to music brought forth a good response from Joan and her lines became freer with more coordinated movements.

In addition, Joan was given intense remedial work in a small group with materials and exercises designed to improve her ability to form letters and to hold the pencil correctly. It was necessary for Joan to use a broad soft pencil and to carefully delineate the space in which she was to make her letters with boxes, lines, etc. Initially, she was taught to make letters with the help of dot cues and colors.

During spelling sessions, Joan responded to an auditory approach. Being a very rhythmical and musical little girl, she also responded well to the use of rhythm instruments (drums, triangle, tambourine) and singing. Her attention span lengthened and the rhythmic beat accompanying spelling served to speed up her oral work and later her written work as well. Difficulties in writing were still apparent and although she was gaining in her ability to form letters and to print, it was not a pleasant task for her. Consequently, much "verbal filibustering" on her part took place in hopes of delaying or postponing altogether that moment when she would really have to write. Colored pencils and chalk were used to fragment parts of letters still difficult for Joan to form. A thick black pencil and reinforced color lines for spatial orientation were necessary. She filled in missing letters, printed words from picture clues, completed sentences in both spelling and English language workbooks.

Music and rhythm played an important part in other areas of her development too. Rhythmic clapping could help her recall rhymes and rhyme words in poetry; it aided in giving her a sense of timing in playing catch with a ball; buttoning and unbuttoning became "more fun." In regular music classes, she was becoming better coordinated in hops, skips, and directional movement (forward, backward, sidewise). Joan learned to manipulate drum sticks and perform drum rhythms, beat a triangle, and clap a castanet.

JOAN'S high interest and good ability in music led to a desire to learn to play the piano. As piano playing required fine finger dexterity and coordination, it would also have some therapeutic value in developing Joan's small muscles in her hands. The diligence was there and very soon Joan was able to move each finger independently, to play octaves with two hands playing together simultaneously, and to form two or three note chords with either hand. Note reading of music was begun in a way which required Joan to write (print) letter names for notes on the music staff.

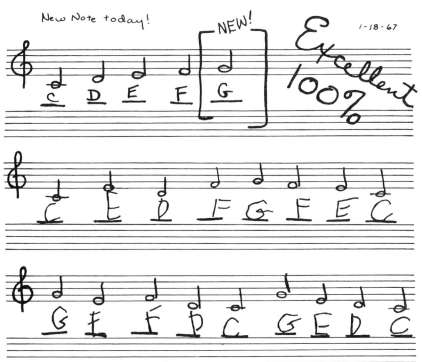

In piano class, the notes were written in a music manuscript book and the child was required to write the name of the note. Colored boxes were first drawn under the note to be named and the child printed the corresponding letter name in the box. On occasion, different colors were used for notes and their respective names to further emphasize the note placement on the staff. The boxes and colors both served to aid the child in locating the note, to visually see the connection between the letter name and note, and to structure the space for the written response. A transfer from boxes for letter names to single lines spaced directly below the notes was made and it was noted that although only a base line served to space letters for notes, a uniform height in letter formation was still being adhered to. Even when lines were omitted, spacing of letters remained accurate as notes gave a visual cue for spacing.

JOAN wanted very much to learn to play the piano by note. This incentive led to a neatly written and quite legible manuscript book. Erasures were at a minimum and letters were uniform in formation and spacing. The correlation between symbols of music (a treble clef sign 𝄞 indicating the starting point at the left; double bar lines ‖ indicating the stopping point or right) aided in reinforcing and clarifying left-to-right orientation.

Comparisons were made between the quality of Joan's written work in the classroom and in the piano class. Her work in a composition book in the classroom often was still illegible. Letters or words were crowded together; or perhaps sentences began in the middle of the page instead of at the left. She was also having difficulty copying correctly from the board. The differences in her writing were so apparent that we decided to try the "musical approach." An individual program of educational therapy was then designed for Joan, employing the same techniques that were used in her piano class.

A music manuscript book became her composition book for handwriting. In the beginning, the format was a melodic line with each note or measure symbolizing an entire word at the top of the page. The second stave of the music paper became the sentence, words, or "song" for Joan to copy. The third stave was Joan's writing line and was structured with colored lines reinforcing top, bottom, and middle for spacing height of letters. The first line of the five-line music staff was reinforced with green, saying, "It's okay to go through if you are a tail letter (*p, y, g*, etc.)"; the third line was reinforced in red, saying, "Stop! unless you are a tall letter"; and the fifth line was reinforced in blue as, "The sky where tall letters reach."

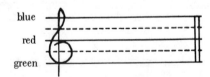

As Joan's tall letters were not quite tall enough and letters such as *a, o, w*, etc., tended to be too large, these color cues and verbal explanations helped to set in her mind what was expected of her printing. As her page was being set up for her, she would respond with the verbal explanation of the color as the color was being used to reinforce a line. Treble clef signs 𝄞 were used on all lines, melodic or word, to structure a starting point. Likewise, double bar lines ‖ as well as periods were used to point out the ending or right side of the page.

The following is a reproduction taken from Joan's manuscript book in handwriting. It shows the format of the page as well as a sample of her handwriting.

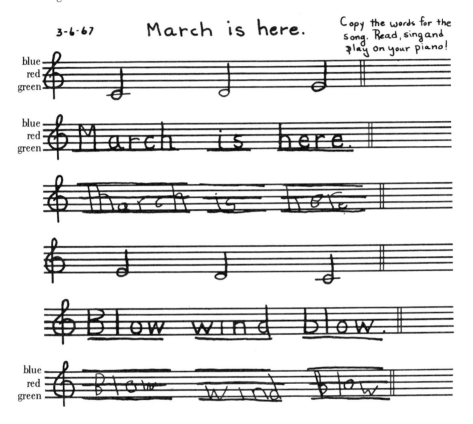

IT WAS extremely important to Joan that each sentence, word, or group of words had a melodic counterpart. The melody not only provided visual cues for word spacing, but also motivation for carrying out the assignment. She would not begin at first until some kind of melody was written. Further incentive was provided by singing or playing the melody before beginning to have Joan write the corresponding words.

Care was taken to use notes (whole notes: ○ ; half notes: 𝅗𝅥 ; quarter notes: ♩) within her note-reading realm so that she could play her "song" for herself at home on her piano. Sentences formed were based on her spelling words, thus giving additional practice in learning to write these words. Sentences were also within her reading vocabulary in order that no difficulty would arise when she played her "song" and sang it to herself later, as she most always did. Notes provided the visual cue for spacing of words and on occasion broken colored lines were also used to space each word. When difficulty$_3$ appeared with spacing of letters within the word, a triplet pattern of notes (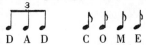) or a series of eighth notes (♪♪♪♪) would be used to emphasize the number of letters in the word and the spacing necessary for each letter. For example:

D A D   C O M E

Joan began to take the same care and show the same interest in writing the words or sentences in her composition manuscript book as she did in writing in her music note-reading manuscript book.

T O ENLARGE the visual range for copying, the format was later changed to a page beginning with music, words to be copied; music line repeated; then Joan's writing line. Finally, the page was set up with music, then Joan's writing line; and the copying was to be done from a speller, reader, or other book; and finally back once again to the chalkboard.

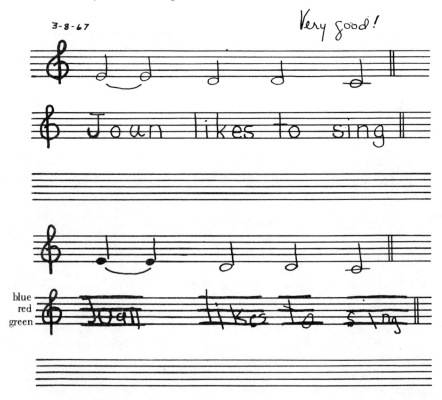

For recall of a spelling word, a sentence and its melody were rewritten on a different page, leaving out the spelling word. From the song, Joan could recall the word and write it in the blank space left for it, then recopy the entire sentence as a whole.

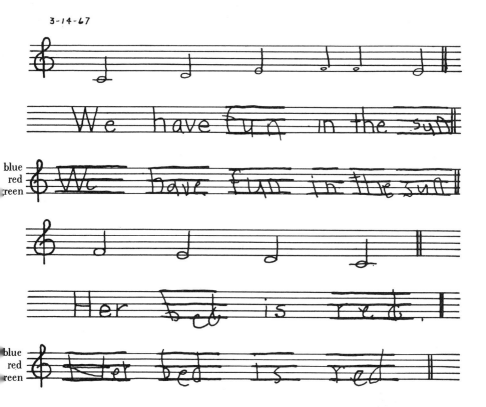

A game, "Find the Mystery Word," in which the clues were notes written on the music staff, was utilized to give practice in printing. Upon being identified, the notes would spell the word.

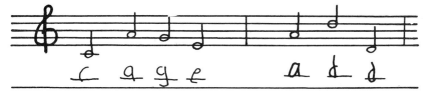

THE INTEREST in writing created by this approach for Joan has begun to carry over in her printing in workbooks and regular composition books. One finds her work better spaced on the page, between the words, and between letters within the word. Letters are better formed and more uniform in size. Joan still benefits from having a reinforced middle line for half-space letters; however, she is able to judge stopping points for both tall and tail letters without reinforced lines.

A musical approach to handwriting has been beneficial to Joan. She is learning to express herself in a written form. Her rhythmical and musical capabilities helped us to lead her to her success in achieving the giant step she has taken in handwriting, thus opening another door in her developmental processes.

E. G. S. has helped me to go.
And now I don't feal so low
Pictograming just brought
tears -
But now it's as easy as
shifting gears -
     by Nathan
        8 th grade

Overburdened Cognitive Processes

George H. Early
Earl J. Heath

L EARNING-DISABLED children have a common characteristic: They tend to intellectualize many tasks, activities, and procedures which could be performed more efficiently at an automatic level. In many situations in which a normal child would respond automatically, the learning-disabled child must deal cognitively with the situation before responding.

N. C. Kephart gives a classic example of overburdened cognitive processes in the case of a ten-year-old boy who was asked to write his name on the chalkboard. [1] In response to this simple demand, the boy first placed his wrist on the board and wrote with finger movements, duplicating as nearly as possible the movements involved in writing with pencil and paper. Each stroke of each letter was made as a separate and distinct operation, with a noticeable pause between strokes. Every teacher and every clinician who deals with learning problems has seen this type of performance at times.

This particular boy, however, gives us a valuable clue to the underlying rea-

sons for this fragmented and agonizing approach to the simple task of writing his name. When he finished, he turned to the examiner and said, "I can write my name. I have memorized the movements." Memorized movements! What he is telling us is that each small portion of each letter requires recall and planning of a specific movement before that small portion can be executed. Moreover, before executing the memorized, fragmented movement associated with any one portion of a letter, he probably must make a mental review of which portions he has already completed, as well as a simultaneous mental forecast of which movement is coming next. Thus, his cognitive processes become overburdened. Too much cognitive attention is required for the movements involved in the act of writing; little, if any, cognitive attention is available for attending to what is being written.

Reflect for a moment upon how you write. Do you dredge up from your memory bank a number of highly specific movements for each letter? Must you recall each movement and plan how you will make that movement before you set pen to paper? Surely not. Undoubtedly you have a "wired in"

[1] Newell C. Kephart, *The Brain-Injured Child in the Classroom* (Chicago, Ill.: National Easter Seal Society for Crippled Children and Adults, 1963).

and highly generalized pattern for writing. When you write, you can bring this pattern into action and the specific movements come automatically. Letters, whole words, even entire phrases, can be summoned forth, and the specific movements will take care of themselves. your cognitive processes are free to deal with the ideas about which you are writing. You do not have to clutter the cognitive channels with cognitive garbage such as the movements involved in producing one insignificant part of one little letter. To the extent that you have developed a generalized movement pattern for writing, your cognitive processes are freed of the burden of dealing with specific movements which should come automatically. You can pay attention to what you are writing, rather than to the movements of writing.

One of Kephart's most far-ranging contributions to education is the concept of the generalized movement pattern. The example cited above is only one small aspect of the implications embodied in this concept. The general principle might be summarized as follows: Cognitive processes should be reserved for matters which are properly at the cognitive level. Conversely, cognitive processes should not be wasted on activities which should unfold automatically. The ultimate aim of developing generalized movement patterns is to relegate automatic functions to automatic levels of the central nervous system — freeing, in the process, the cognitive levels for their proper task of dealing with cognitive matters.

When generalized movement patterns have been achieved the child is freed of many blocks to learning. Cognitive attention can focus upon the goal of movement instead of being diverted into wasteful attending to movements *per*

se. Movement, and activity in general, is then available for exploration of the environment, for becoming an agent whereby information from the child's surroundings is received, processed, compared with previous experience, and integrated as a meaningful part of his total fund of knowledge. The child who must deal cognitively with the movements incidental to traversing his surroundings inevitably is impoverished by a corresponding loss of meaningful encounter with the world in which he operates.

IF ONE grants the fundamental position just presented, a major educational goal emerges: Many children must be helped to develop generalized movement patterns so that many blocks to learning may be removed. Activities which are preeminently automatic must be removed from the cognitive levels and planted firmly in the automatic levels of functioning. The cognitive processes must be relieved of cumbersome burdens and set free for the exciting task of true learning.

How may generalized movement patterns be developed in children who lack them? Normally, one should first attend to the development of overall and fairly gross motor activity. The child's general motor development should be such that he moves, typically, in a flexible and coordinated fashion. He should be able to make selective and controlled use of each body part through the entire range of movement of which that part is capable. Further, the individual parts should be capable of an equally wide range of flexible and combined movements, where parts work together in solving a variety of motor problems. A child develops such generalized movement patterns at this gross level through numerous experiences in which he employs a great variety of specific movements in performing the same or a similar task. In doing the same task in many different ways, he thus develops a generalized pattern of movement for that task, rather than a narrow set of isolated and specific movement. [2] The development of these overall generalized body-movement patterns usually should precede attempts to promote development of higher-level generalized movement patterns such as those involved in writing.

In the case of the ten-year-old boy who had "memorized the movements" for writing his name, one would first attend to developing an overall pattern of flexible and coordinated movements, assuming this pattern was not present at the outset. It then would be in order to begin remedial activities aimed at developing a generalized movement pattern for writing.

At the Achievement Center for Children (Purdue University), an approach that is frequently employed is a variation of the Fernald method, the major modifications of which were developed by Rhoda Wharry.[3] Cursive writing is employed exclusively. If the child does not know the cursive alphabet, it is taught to him, beginning with the letters that are easiest to form and progressing to those that are more difficult. If he already knows the cursive alphabet, the method is used for teaching him spelling words and those words which give him trouble in reading.

At first, large-size cursive writing is used (six to eight inches high) the letters becoming progressively smaller as the child becomes more competent. Thus, the initial stages involve gross arm movements exclusively, and the error of developing fine motor skills ahead of gross motor abilities is avoided.

In teaching a word, the therapist first makes a large cursive copy of the word. The child then traces the word several times, saying the sound (or sometimes the name) of each letter as he traces the letter, and sustaining the sound during the entire period the hand is tracing that letter. Synchrony of voice, eye, and hand is emphasized, and the therapist works for smooth and rhythmical arm movements.

When the child's tracing performance is fairly adequate, he is asked to copy the word several times, referring to the tracing for help as he needs it. When he no longer needs to look back at the tracing, he is asked to write the word from memory. A large flashcard is made for each word learned in this way, with the word written in cursive on one side and in manuscript on the other. The flashcards are used to check for retention, with words that are not retained being treated as new words to be learned.

Generalized movement patterns for writing are promoted in several ways by the large-cursive-writing program. Writing is done in different body positions: standing at the chalkboard, seated at the table, seated on the floor, on hands and knees on the floor, and in any other position the therapist can devise. Methods of tracing are varied: with the finger, in the air, with chalk, with crayon, with pencil, etc. Writing materials are also varied: chalk with

---

[2] For a full treatment of generalized movement patterns, see Newell C. Kephart, *The Slow Learner in the Classroom* (Columbus, Ohio: Charles E. Merrill, 1960), and *Learning Disability: An Educational Adventure* (West Lafayette, Ind.: Kappa Delta Pi Press, 1968).

[3] Rhoda E. Wharry, "Perceptual-Motor Generalizations and Remedial Reading." Unpublished doctoral dissertation (Lafayette, Ind.: Purdue University, 1969).

chalkboard, or paper with crayon, felt marker, pencil, etc. The position of the writing surface is changed frequently: vertical, horizontal, and various degrees of slant.

W ITH all of these variations, the common task of writing is accomplished. The variations, however, free the child from the necessity of employing a rigid and restricted skill and permit him instead to develop a general and an internalized pattern for writing. Different muscle groups perform the task; different tactual-kinesthetic feedback come from employing a variety of writing materials. Rather than relying on a highly specific set of memorized movements, the child develops a generalized pattern, and when this occurs there is often a corresponding release of cognitive processes for their proper functioning.

Some Notes on the Teaching of Handwriting

Alice Russell McKenna

———————————————

THE TEACHING of legible handwriting is, of course, an essential and even hallowed aspect of the school curriculum, but it is an even more indispensable part of the remedial training program for children with Specific Language Disability. Indeed, the development of the ability to form letters correctly and to link them fluidly into words is basic to the kinesthetic process involved in the special training for facility in word recognition and spelling used with these children. The suggestions set forth in this article, therefore, are presented with the particular needs of remedial students in mind. They are equally applicable to the teaching of handwriting in the regular classroom.

Since underdevelopment of the visual-motor skills is usually a characteristic of students with expressive language difficulty — most immediately evident in their poorly-formed and irregular script — some basic training in exercises designed to foster eye-hand coordination is fundamental to improvement of the writing process.

We begin in a "large" way — that is to say, with large movements of the whole body, and then of the writing hand — in space:

Body: Exercises to establish firm concepts of left-and-rightness, and of directionality.

Hand: Left-to-right; top-to-bottom; describing circles, ovals, squares, rectangles, triangles, verticals, horizontals, loops. We move to the chalkboard: wet sponge making the large shapes, with perhaps a few flourishes of curlicues and arabesques — delightful! Make it a good large sponge, for kneading, and squeezing, and enjoying. Wet the chalkboard and use large kindergarten chalks or the broad side of regular chalk for making sweeping forms on the elegantly smooth surface. (The board will have to be washed carefully after this procedure, or it will be peopled by permanent ghosts.) The teacher's hand guides and directs the formation of these shapes, and eventually, of numbers and letters. The child looks, names the shape with the teacher as he makes it, feels it in the motion of his hand and arm. He looks away from the board, naming, making, feeling, as the teacher guides his hand, and thus he begins to know in his bones, the shapes of the symbols he is working on.

Much guided practice is given first, slowly and carefully, and gradually the child begins to feel free and sure, and even daring enough to try the experiment of looking away from the board, and forming the designs himself, freely and easily, without having to give close visual attention to the process. Later, when he is working on paper at the desk, he will experiment in this way again, as a necessary change from closely-watched writing.

Big sheets of unlined paper, perhaps smooth-surfaced butcher's paper; good crayons; felt pens; long rolls of colored shiny shelf paper; aluminum foil; wet sand in a tray; fine sandpaper; flocked paper; last night's evening paper and a paint brush; finger paints — all are helpful media for the child just learning to write or for the remedial student getting a fresh start.

Just holding a pencil properly can be a problem, so there need to be hand and finger exercises as well: grasping and releasing; finger-tapping on a desk, firmly and rhythmically; the lifting and lowering of designated fingers on command; picking up jackstraws or toothpicks or matches; turning a stiff doorknob, or a key in a lock; sorting cards; playing jacks or marbles; shuffling cards; "playing the piano" on a desk, with hands arched properly and fingers pressing down firmly; manipulating puzzles; handling wooden letter and number forms with eyes closed, as an aid in identification; pinching up confetti from a rug; kneading plasticene; wringing out a wet cloth or sponge; holding chalk in the correct overhand position and a pencil in comfortable writing position — the list is endless. Rich source-material for the development of eye-hand coordination may be found in

the books by Helene Durbrow,[1] Marianne Frostig,[2] G. N. Getman,[3] and Newell Kephart.[4]

Tracing felt, flocked, or wooden letters and numbers with the fingers; tracing inset designs in templates or formboards with a pencil, helps to develop an accurate feeling for shapes. Tracing over pictures in a coloring book, simple embroidery designs, or clearly detailed pictures from a discarded reader can be helpful. Tracing large numbers and letters on chalkboard, chart paper, heavy cardboard, in blocks of clay or wax, and on lined paper forms another step in the writing process.

And here we come to the knotty problem of the type of script to be used for tracing and copying. Shall it be the "printed manuscript" form widely taught in the first and second grades, or shall it be cursive, or "running" script, to which children usually graduate in the third grade? Cursive writing is the script of choice for all grade levels, from the remedial standpoint, because it presents freedom from confusion of similar letter-forms (*b* and *d*; *p* and *q*; *n* and *h*, for example) and because its continuous flowing motion tends to obviate letter reversals in writing. The clinician will wish, therefore, to proceed with teaching or retraining in the cursive form. If one is working with a first

---

[1]Helene C. Durbrow, *Learning to Write* (Cambridge, Massachusetts: Educators Publishing Service, 1968).

[2]M. Frostig and D. Horne, *Teacher's Guide. The Frostig Program for the Development of Visual Perception* (Chicago, Illinois: Follett Publishing Co., 1964).

[3]G. N. Getman and E. R. Kane, *The Physiology of Readiness* (Minneapolis, Minnesota: P.A.S.S., Inc., 1964).

[4]Newell C. Kephart, *The Slow Learner in the Classroom* (Columbus, Ohio: Charles E. Merrill Books, Inc., 1960).

or second grader who is learning the manuscript form at school, it will be necessary to consult with his classroom teacher and come to an agreement about the matter. Many teachers agree to the child's early introduction to cursive writing in the clinic laboratory, and the child himself enjoys learning this "advanced" skill. Sometimes, however, it may be important psychologically that the child continue to adhere to the manuscript form being used by his classmates. A kind of compromise can be effected, then, by teaching the "joined manuscript" form at the clinic. In this form the strokes are concluded with a small, flowing link or "join" to the next printed letter. Here is a comparison of the two methods:

Manuscript

Joined Manuscript

Teaching the formation of letters in related sequence of execution is important. Usually this pattern is followed: (I have substituted *qu* for simple *q.*)

a c d g o qu

l t h b k f i j p

e r s n m u w

v y x z

In forming these letters, it is important to keep the pencil *on the page,* to facilitate smoothness of execution. For example, in making *b,* start at the top, bring the stroke down to the line, keep the pencil *on the paper* and bring it back up along the downstroke, then around, out and in again to the bottom of the downstroke, and out in the short join, or link. In making *d,* start as with *c;* around and out to the left, down to the line, and up, *pencil on the paper,* then down over the upstroke to the line again, ending in the short link stroke.

While the use of the "joined manuscript" form is not foolproof for the child with reversal tendencies, it can be made workable.

With students who are already familiar with cursive writing, the remedial training will consist in helping them work for greater ease in making the alphabet forms they have already been taught in the classroom, and the agile clinician will prepare the individual practice materials with a weather-eye out for whatever variation in alphabet style the student is accustomed to, helping him to form these letters correctly and easily. Variations in the system of page guidelines need not cause great difficulty, as long as there is a guideline above to mark the boundary for capital letters, and a double line beneath it to keep all the small letters marching along in orderly fashion. Guidelines to indicate correct slant may be superimposed on the page, as well.

It is helpful to have several kinds of lined practice paper on hand, with wide and narrow spaces between lines, to adjust to individual needs in the matter of comfortable functioning in space. Students enjoy experimenting with different types of paper and writing implements, and will bring to the creative task of handwriting a rather astonishing amount of enthusiasm!

Where it seems desirable to modify the cursive style for greater ease in execution, an alphabet something like this might be useful:

The study of alphabets is usually fascinating to students, who enjoy comparing scripts as listed in a dictionary or encyclopedia, or the samples given in books on printing and type-faces. Often older students, who might tend to resent spending all the time really needed for practice, will become absorbed in copying or inventing interesting alphabetic designs. Comparisons of styles used in old manuscripts and in documents, evaluation charts, and commercial workbooks is always interesting and often suggestive of new techniques. *New Yorker* readers will be fascinated by the wonderfully complicated designs of Saul Steinberg, executed with magnificent flourishes of penmanship. The very handsome "italic script" is well worth their investigating and experimenting with, too. See George Thomson for a detailed exposition of this method.[5]

With our preliminary coordination training established and referred to for continual reinforcement as needed, and the student ready and eager to work with paper and pencil at the desk, we now provide teacher-made models for tracing. There will be solid-line alphabets on a forward slant, and solid-line alphabets on a backward slant, for children who find this direction more comfortable. Here again, some experimenting may be in order, for not everyone finds the customary forward slant suitable, or convenient, or expressive of his own developing style. Dorothy Emerson provides clear letter-samples for both forward and backward slant writing practice.[6] Boundary lines which keep the letters properly aligned on the page will be clearly delineated. Anna Gillingham has an excellent discussion of handwriting methods in her valuable Remedial Training manual.[7]

The student is taught from the beginning to seat himself in correct posture, feet on floor or a footstool, with paper slanted to the left at a 45 degree angle for the right-handed child, and to the right at the same angle for the left-handed child. He should sit so that the elbows come comfortably to the surface of the desk, with shoulders in a relaxed position, the subdominant hand resting at the top of the page, the writing hand holding the pencil easily but firmly. He may be taught how to position his paper correctly by having him place his arms on the desk with fingers of both hands barely meeting, so that an even triangle is formed by his forearms and trunk. The position of the paper, then, conforms to and is an extension of, the right hand and arm for the right-handed child, and the left hand and arm for the left-handed child. The paper may be taped to the desk to ensure its staying in the correct position. A desk top slanted at an eleven degree tilt is preferable to a flat writing surface. See Luella Cole[8] and Mildred Plunkett[9] for correct teaching procedure with left-handed children. Parents who spend hours drilling the arms-off-the-table routine

[7]A. Gillingham and B. Stillman, *Remedial Training for Children with Specific Disability in Reading, Spelling, and Penmanship* (Cambridge, Massachusetts: Educators Publishing Service, 1960).

[8]Luella Cole, *Handwriting for Left-Handed Children* (Bloomington, Illinois: Public School Publishing Co., 1955).

[9]Mildred B. Plunkett, *A Writing Manual for Teaching the Left-Handed* (Cambridge, Massachusetts: Educators Publishing Service, 1954, 1967).

[5]George Thomson, *Better Handwriting* (Great Britain: Penguin Books, Ltd., 1957. Catalogue number, PP 96.

[6]Dorothy Emerson, *Help Yourself to Better Handwriting* (Cambridge, Massachusetts: Educators Publishing Service, 1954).

into their young without observing significant change in their dining deportment should be pleased to know that this particular lesson has been, nevertheless, only too well absorbed. Unfortunately the teacher has to spend about the same amount of time reminding students that the arm must be *on* the table for writing!

The student's writing-life now centers on tracing, tracing, and more tracing, with simultaneous naming (or sounding) of each letter as it is being traced. Lower-case and capital letters; numbers; difficult letter-combinations; words; short sentences, form the sequence of exercises. The teacher watches carefully, noticing any difficulties with starting points, stroke direction, and the like, and provides clues on the page, or a guiding hand, or a red stylus trailing the direction on the page before the child's pencil, or voiced directions, as guidance. Children who find it difficult to stay on the line to be traced may need to have the clear, underlying image strongly outlined by the teacher to provide firm boundaries. Interesting variations in media for this process

can be successive colors of chalk at the board or of crayons and pencils at the desk, as the child goes over and over his first tracings.

Pencils for young children should be the large beginners' variety; these are often useful for older students, too. Standard pencils of medium lead may be encircled with a broad cushion of rubber bands at the point of grasp, for the child who tends to hold the pencil too tensely, or at the base of the finger tip to prevent grasping the pencil too close to the point. Ball point pens can be a problem if the point is too fine or the ink supply seems too uncertain or meager. Some careful evaluation is necessary here. Felt pens or laundry marking pens are useful if the ink flows freely. A good fountain pen with a comfortable nib is excellent.

The first models for tracing would show a single letter to be traced several times on a page set up according to the system dearest to one's own heart in regard to margins and placement of name and date. Perhaps it would look something like this:

Ann Smith   *May 5, 1970*

a a   a a   a a

a a   a a   a a

a a   a a   a a

The important thing is to start the child off on the right track regarding acceptable form for written work well placed on the page, properly signed, and dated in full. Children need to be taught from the beginning to aim at the production of polished work in each area of academic life. While we receive their every writing effort with loving appreciation and compliment each achievement with stars or seals or congratulatory notations, we must still keep bringing them forward gently into the accomplishment of truly beautiful written work of a high order.

At the end of each lesson the completed papers will be carefully reviewed with the student, who may then insert them into his ring notebook or paper binder for safekeeping. A paper punch will be a necessity here — either the small hand variety, excellent for finger exercise, or the large, office type. (This is where you get the confetti to pick off the rug!)

The long period of carefully supervised tracing interspersed with copying and practicing on one's own, is exceedingly beneficial. It means a lot of preliminary work by the classroom teacher in preparing practice-forms, but as long as her writing arm holds out and the duplicating machine provides good, clear copies, she can amass enough working material to last quite a long time. She will, of course, do much careful demonstration at the board before the class settles down to its work — the children accompanying her by tracing in the air or on their desks — and then be free to move around the room and give the necessary individual help. The clinician, working on a one-to-one basis, can prepare the practice forms as needed, as the child observes the careful formation of letters while the teacher writes.

Copying from the board a prepared paper or an alphabet model, writing to dictation, and writing freely on one's own, form still other exercises in the writing process. The child will have absorbed, after all his preliminary practice, the idea of the required system for letter-form, word-spacing, and page format, and he should begin to practice the correct use of capitals, spelling, and punctuation, as he writes short sentences. These may be dictated by the teacher or be of his own composition. He may also wish to dictate sentences, stories, short book reports, or social letters to the teacher, who will write them down for him to copy.

False starts, erasures, and smudges are inevitable in the beginning, and may be for a long time to come. Too strict an interpretation of standards on either the teacher's or student's part is frustrating all around, so we happily settle for what the earnest young hand has written, pointing out improvements over previous performance, and tactfully indicating the areas in which more care is needed. Sometimes it is best to drop the writing process for a time and to concentrate on the exercises exclusively, particularly when the child's ambition is outrunning his present capacity. On the other hand, the child who has developed real writing facility, but has grown careless in performance, may profit from using a pencil from which the eraser has been removed, or from being required to do the work over again!

By this time the writing notebook or binder is very plump indeed. How interesting it is to watch the child review his work and make comparisons between early and recent achievement! (Here one often has to help him preserve respect for the early work. It may not be up to his present standards, but it was most carefully and honestly done, and quite right for the child he was a few months ago.) And how delightful to overhear a child remarking of another in his group, "Charlie *really* knows how to make *g*'s and *j*'s now. They're great!" Or, "Hey, I made up a new finger exercise. Can we give it a whirl?"

And what are the rewards for all this earnest effort and long, hard practice? Papers displayed with pride on bulletin boards as each new step is taken; a handwriting certificate complete with gold seals and a solemn commendatory statement of demonstrated progress — of course! (One little boy gave his *teacher* a diploma, wrought with painstaking care and tied with a ribbon, after he had laboriously earned his own certificate!) But the real boon is the tremendous feeling of satisfaction which comes from serious personal effort, culminating in results which both satisfy one's own developing taste and dazzle the bystander.

The older student, now committed to the proposition that legible handwriting, neatly organized papers, and careful attention to spelling, grammar, and punctuation bring dividends of their own in the form of improved grades, is equally heartened. He knows that handwriting is a very personal expression of creativity, over and above its practical value as a means of communicating his ideas, and that this skill needs all the cultivation of which he is capable. And the student who has really suffered over his disability in this very important area of the language arts finds his frustrations melting away as his handwriting begins to convey beautifully and clearly the precious burden of his thoughts.

In every case, there is the triumphant glow of personal joy in mastery of a valued skill — and this, I believe, is the very best reward a teacher could possibly ask, for her children or for herself.

Cursive Writing: An Analytical Approach

Martha Serio

SINCE CHILDREN with learning disabilities often have difficulty in visual perception and/or motor coordination, both of which are essential to the act of handwriting, it appears that teachers must take into consideration resources for aiding the child in these areas. Descriptions of methods and materials which are useful for teaching the child with learning disabilities in the art of handwriting are discussed by William M. Cruickshank and by Alfred A. Strauss and Laura E. Lehtinen.[1] Some of these techniques have been used successfully in special classes. The intent of this article is not to review these writings, but to re-emphasize some of their major points and add to the teacher's information. The composite of these ideas would not necessarily "fit" any one child's liabilities but should be used discriminately for specific problems.

Most educators seem to be in agreement that the child with learning disabilities should be taught cursive rather than manuscript writing. The following reasons are cited:

• *The rhythm involved in cursive writing lends itself to a more effici-*

[1] See references.

ent use of movement. By way of contrast, manuscript seems to promote jerky movements which should be avoided. In addition, the smoother flow of movement in cursive writing seems to reinforce tactile learning and enable the child to hold the letter and/or word together.

• *Proper spacing is aided in the writing of words.* Single letters, written alone, have an extra "swing" which aids in setting them apart. The connecting stroke serves to separate letters written together. With practice the spacing between letters becomes more even and helps to eliminate the convergence or the discontinuity of letters within a word. This feature also aids in holding words together as units.

• *A single method approach eliminates the problem of retraining.* It has been observed that a child who has previously been taught manuscript has difficulty in changing to cursive. This may be especially important to a child with perceptual handicap since many of them display rigidity and difficulty in establishing a new mental image.

• *The forms of individual letters*

65

in cursive writing seem to be more independent of confusion due to directionality. There is still a chance for confusion of similar letters in cursive writing, but not for the same reason as manuscript. It would appear that confusion of direction is the important cause for the confusion of similar letters in manuscript, such as *b-d, p-q, m-w,* etc.

IN RECENT YEARS numerous articles have been written concerning techniques for the "training" of directionality. If one can accept this assumption, then it could follow that developmentally the training of directionality is a prerequisite to teaching of manuscript writing. I am questioning the "transfer of learning." Could not transfer of learning be a separate entity and a specific disability for the child with learning disabilities? It thus becomes a disability that is not easily, if ever, fully retrained. It has been observed that, for unknown reasons, when a child uses manuscript he will revert to a reversal pattern under stress.

The differences in similar letters in cursive writing are not determined by differences according to direction, but are different in appearance by addition or deletion of lines. The reproduction or coding of language in cursive form therefore seems particularly necessary for the child who has a directional problem since there is no need to delay the skill of writing because of directional disabilities which may or may not be ultimately "retrained."

Readiness Materials.

STRAUSS, and later Cruickshank advocated the use of readiness exercises on beginning writing. Strauss wrote:

> Our aim is to encourage writing readiness, assuming that the

learning of writing depends as much upon the psychological factors of visual perception as upon the maturation of neuro-muscular coordination. (p. 184)

I believe that many of the methods used even now are still based upon assumption! From our experience, the use of readiness materials are, or only can be, useful if they are designed to train a specific problem. The cursive letters are made up of parts which when put together form a whole (Gestalt). The readiness material will then be designed of actual lines that are the parts of a completed cursive letter. For example:

Using this attack, the teacher can construct readiness materials as advocated by the cited authors.

• The "direction lines" can be made with a felt pen on tag boards with various colors, beginning with two and adding colors for more complex figures. The act of picking up and using one color and then putting it down before proceeding with another color to follow through in making the next part reinforces the relationships of the parts of letters that comprise the whole figure.

• The child may copy on tracing paper or acetate covers with crayons, finally using one color.

• After the tracing exercise, the child may draw the same figures on a plain sheet of paper which at first has lines drawn on it and is later folded to insure proper spacing and size.

• The number of lines is geared to the individual child's needs, beginning with simple exercises and then progressing on to the more complex, and moving from larger to smaller lines and figures.

• The beginning movement for one-space letters can be divided into one of the following three movements:

$$\circ \quad \cup \quad \subset$$

Using these lines for readiness activities, the teacher will be able to begin teaching one-space letters in the group that is easiest for the child to complete. The two- and three-space letters are taught later. The readiness activities and actual writing are in reality taught simultaneously. Using this technique the letters could be grouped accordingly:

i e r s u w / t / j p

m n x v / y

a c o / d g q

b h l k / f

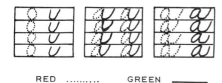

RED .... GREEN ———

Cursive Writing.

• The circumference of the instrument used for writing may vary with each child's needs. If needed, a small rubber ball forced to the point of grasp will provide a larger surface for the child who has difficulty with control of small objects.

• A wristlet, usually weighted with sand, will hold the wrist in the proper position. It is also useful for the ambidextrous child, as the weight can be placed on the wrist of the dominant side.

• The spacing or width of lines is determined according to each child's needs. In recent years, numerous types of writing paper have become available. They vary not only as to various space structures, but as to number of lines. (A list of materials and where they may be obtained can be found at the end of this article.) If the child is unable to stay within thin writing lines, a wider line may be drawn with a felt pen, ultimately returning to a narrow line. If the child has difficulty starting on the proper line, different colors can be used to emphasize top and bottom. In order to add variety to the task, and to avoid rigidity, the color cues may be changed, finally returning to one color.

• The size of the writing paper is also an important factor to consider. The paper must be placed at the proper angle and be within range of the eyes.

FOR MANY YEARS, the conventional writing paper used by beginners has been wide. Some children with writing disabilities tend to have a great deal of difficulty remembering to move the paper. As the child writes from left to right, the letters toward the right side of the page become progressively worse in construction. This problem can be avoided by giving the child a narrow paper — perhaps no more than four inches wide.

I recall a seven-year-old boy who could write only one letter at a time. He could not place letters across the page, nor could he move down the page. He was given a piece of paper just large enough for one letter and then he stapled these onto a plain sheet of paper. By this means he was able to do his half sheet of writing each day.

Thus, the methods, the length of assignment, the design or structure of the paper and the presentation of letters are geared to the child's disability. It is completely unrealistic to approach all children with any one method. The teaching approaches are designed for the child; the child is not designed for the method.

WRITING MATERIALS

- Pencil paper, green tint, 2″ ruling, 8″ x 10½″ ruled both sides long way. No. 150170. No. 0-A Paper.
- Pencil paper, green tint, 1″ ruling, 8″ x 10½″ ruled both sides long way. No. 150180. No. 1-A Paper.
- Cursive Trac-A-Bit Sets. Six complete alphabets of capital letters and six alphabets of lower-case letters and numerals to be used with grease pencils that can be erased.

The above items are available from Zaner-Bloser, 612 North Park Street, Columbus, Ohio 43215

- White primary pencil paper, No. 605, 9″ x 12 ″. One-half inch alternate rule long way. One inch blank space every third line.
- White primary pencil paper, No. 319, 8″ x 10″. Three-eighths inch alternate rule long way.
- White primary pencil paper, No. 601, 9″ x 12″. Three-eighths inch alternate rule long way.
- White primary pencil paper, No. 101R, 9″ x 12″. One-half inch long way. Every third line heavy red lines.
- White primary pencil paper, No. 102R, 9″ x 12″. One-fourth inch long way. Every fourth line heavy red lines.

- Green tint sight saving (fourth grade), No. 444, 8″ x 10½″. Three-eighths inch short way, one side; alternate 5/32 − 7/32 one side.
- Green tint primary pencil paper, No. 333X, 8″ x 10½″. One-fourth inch alternate rule long way one side, one-half inch rule long way one side.

The above supplies are available from the Dobson-Evans Company, 1100 West Third Avenue, Columbus, Ohio 43212.

- Imaginary Line Handwriting Beginning Cursive Book.

This aid may be obtained from the Steck-Vaugh Company in Austin, Texas.

REFERENCES

Cruickshank, William M. *A Teaching Method for Brain-Injured and Hyperactive Children.* Syracuse, N.Y.: Syracuse University Press, 1961.

——————— (ed.). *The Teacher of Brain-Injured Children: A Discussion of the Bases for Competency.* Syracuse, N.Y. Syracuse University Press, 1966.

——————— . *The Brain-Injured Child in Home, School, and Community.* Syracuse, N.Y. — Syracuse University Press, 1967.

Strauss, Alfred A., and Laura E. Lehtinen. *Psychopathology and Education of the Brain Injured Child.* New York: Grune and Stratton, 1947.

Handwriting and Vision

Ernest J. Kahn

———————◆•◆———————

FOR MANY years we have known of the deleterious effect of improper posture while reading and writing on our physical structure and physical conditions. The monumental work of Darell Boyd Harmon,[1] which connects the learning environment of the classroom, its physical attributes of illuminations, desk construction, and relative positions in the classroom to spine curvature and visual anomalies, leaves very little unsaid. Yet, today, over twenty years later, we are still beset by more or less the very same problems.[2] In the fall of 1967, I began to photograph children with learning problems while they were doing the copy form test, because as a group I had noticed that they demonstrated such poor posture during the test.[3]

After a short time, I started taking pictures of every child and some adults while they were doing the writing test, because a pattern was emerging. It seemed that the prevalence of improper head posture and improper finger grips of the pencil was much greater than I had ever considered possible. I will leave the statistical correlation to some future researcher. It suffices for me to document some of the abberations of the writing act so that members of all professions working with learning disabilities may be alerted to the nature of the problem.

The association of pencil grip to various visually related problems came to my awareness because of constant repetition of the following during copy form testing.

· Practically all nearsighted children held their pencil no more than a quarter of an inch from the tip.

· Almost all children with learning difficulty exhibited some form of bizarre pencil grip and fine motor incoordination.

In all instances of improper pencil grip, the fingers intercepted the line of sight from the pencil tip to the eye if the head was in a proper position. Therefore, the children and adults all brought their heads to the side and/or

---

[1] Harmon, Darell Boyd. *The Coordinated Classroom,* Austin, Texas. A monograph published by the American Seating Company 1948, Rev. 1951.

[2] Pierce, J. R. Nearpoint Visual Performance and Electrophysiological Changes as a Function of Opitcal, Postural and Distance Variables. Research Report and in OEP papers 1967-68, Indiana College of Optometry.

[3] A modification of the Winterhaven Lions Research Foundation. *Perceptual Forms Test and Training Materials.* Winterhaven, Florida, 1965.

closer to the page so that they could see what they were writing. The basis for this lesson is remarkably well illustrated in a booklet by Luella Cole,[4] which delineates the problem of the left-handed writer. Miss Cole shows the evolution of the left-hand hook as a solution of the pen, hand, writing angle, and head posture problem.

The following unposed photographs illustrate the problems.

From the point of view of head posture, there is very little difference, if any, between the underachiever and the myopic developmental problem. In the case of myopia, I find the short pencil grip to be a concomitant of reading too close in a poor light, in bed, and while lying on the floor.

As previously mentioned, the near visual stress in the underachiever, who writes with his head close to the page and who holds the pencil improperly, occurs as a concomitant of poor fine motor coordination. This poor fine motor coordination frequently has its basis in poor gross motor coordination or some other block to proper fine hand motor control. It follows, from classical optometric thought, that any child who endeavors to write at four to eight inches is working two to three times as hard with his focusing system compared to the focusing required at the normal distance of 13 inches. This alone would serve as one logical explanation of why these children, who were not endowed with the hereditary myopic tendency, have a nearpoint learning problem.

It is my opinion that in order to restore most of these children to successful learning habits, and at the same time preclude the myopic pattern in

the school environment, proper use of paper and pencil is mandatory. The three parts of proper writing are as follows:

1. *Proper body posture:* The writing surface should be approximately at elbow height and the head at the Harmon distance (13 to 16 inches).

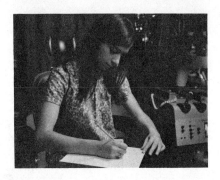

2. *Proper paper angle:* The edges of the page should parallel the direction of the writing forearm for both right and left-handed individuals.

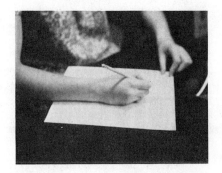

3. *Proper pencil grip:* The pencil should not be held too tightly, with the thumb and index finger about one to one and one-half inches from the writing tip. Left-handed children

---

[4]Cole, Luella. *Handwriting for Left-Handed Children.* Bobbs-Merrill Co.: Indianapolis, Indiana, 1955.

should hold the pencil a little longer than right-handed children to give more seeing room.

The procedure of gripping the pencil is practiced using the *OK* sign as a starting posture from which to go to a relaxed writing pose.

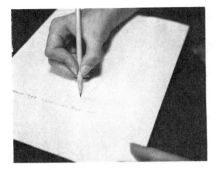

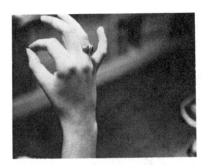

In order to instruct and retrain some of these children in new hand-eye coordination skills, which affects their handwriting, I have evolved certain instructions. To remind them of the proper position on a pencil, I recommend putting a rubber band on the end of the pen or pencil. Better yet is the Grip-Erase. This remarkable triangular, soft plastic gripper slides on the pencil quite easily. It relaxes the fingers and the hand while writing. The three smooth surfaces form support for the thumb, index finger, and side of the middle finger.[5]

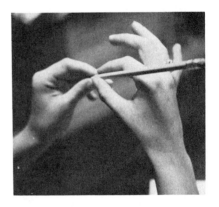

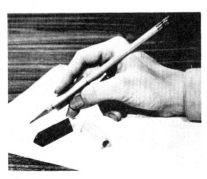

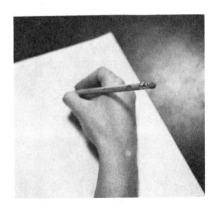

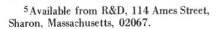

5 Available from R&D, 114 Ames Street, Sharon, Massachusetts, 02067.

The procedure outlined above sounds very simple, and is very simple, if the instruction takes place before

71

ILLUSTRATIONS OF IMPROPER PENCIL GRIP

THUMB TUCKER

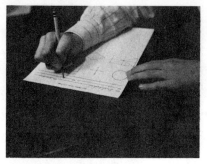

1. David 16—Hyperopia—
   Poor Achiever

THUMB TUCKER

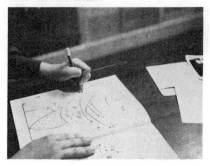

2. Richard 11—Posture—
   Near Point Problem

THUMB TUCKER

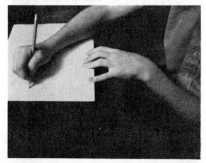

3. Kathy 13—Slow Progressive Myopia

FINGER BENDER & TENSION

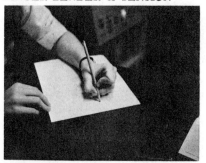

4. Chris 10—Myopia

INDEX FINGER AVOIDANCE

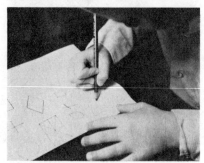

5. Gerald 7.6—Learning to Write
   and Read Problem

GROSS FINGER TENSION

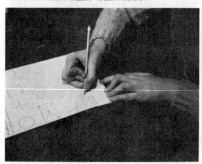

6. Barbara—Myopia

AWKWARD LEFT HAND
GRIPPER

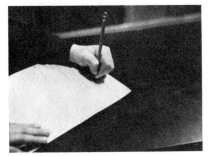

7. Nancy 11–Slow Learner–Aniso

SHORT PENCIL GRIPPER

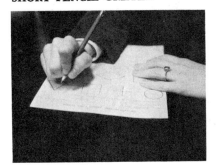

9. Debbie 14–Myopia OD

THUMB AVOIDER

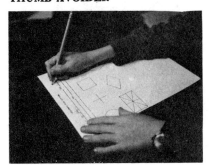

11. Randy 13–Tired Eyes

THUMB TUCKER
FINGER BENDER

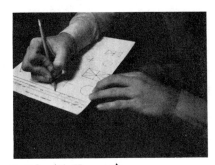

8. John 17–Hyperopia–
Slow in School

INDEX FINGER TUCKER

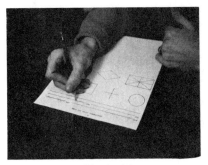

10. Dennis 19–Handwriting
and Drawing Difficulties

THUMB AVOIDER

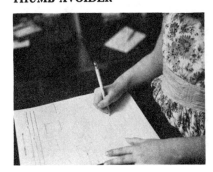

12. Janet 8–Prog. Myopia

ILLUSTRATIONS OF POOR POSTURE
WITH POOR PENCIL GRIP

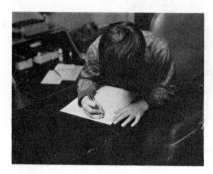

13. Kevin 6—Hyperactive—Hyperope Esotrope

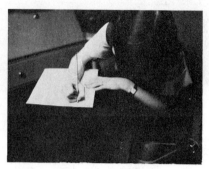

14. June—Short Pencil—Poor Grip

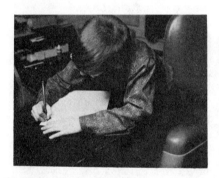

15. David 9-6—Hyperopia, Reading Problem

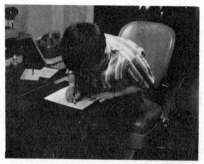

16. Andrew 7—Incipient Myopia

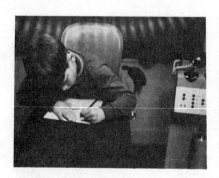

17. Jeff 7-7—Learning Problem Low Hyperope

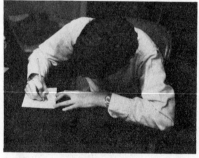

18. Leo 14—Near Performance— Prob.—Hyperopia

the age of seven. It becomes progressively harder for a child to change at a later age from what has become an accustomed, automatic, unconscious habit, which has had many years of strong daily reenforcement. Nevertheless, I have had success, even with some fourteen-year-old children, where the motivation to overcome a particular difficulty was commensurately strong.

I have illustrated a relationship between poor pencil grip, poor posture, and certain perceptual visual problems. A method of retraining has been suggested, and I feel that proper handwriting and use of a pencil is mandatory for comprehensive rehabilitation of myopia and learning difficulty problems.

This article originally appeared in the *Journal of the American Optometric Association* (February 1969) Volume 40, number 2, and is included here with the permission of the author and editor.

A hobby is something you like to do in your spare time. Some people like to fix cars and some people like to work on their stamp collections. I like to watch television because you learn lots of things on it.

Roger

Some Practical Considerations in the Teaching of Handwriting

Diana Hanbury King

KINESTHETIC reinforcement is the *sine qua non* of all successful remedial work, and the importance of correct training in handwriting cannot be overemphasized. Kinesthetic patterns, once learned, are more firmly embedded than those of any other sense. He who has once learned to ride a bicycle or a horse, to skate or ski, or to use a typewriter, will not lose the skill, even after years of disuse. Unlike visual or auditory stimuli, which feed into both hemispheres of the brain, handwriting is a unilateral cerebral activity and serves to establish and reinforce dominance, the lack of which is related to difficulty in any area of language.

Writing is often the first step in learning to read, for it is only when the dyslexic child begins to feel the shape of the letters that the symbols begin to stick in his memory. In the more severe cases of dyslexia, remedial work often fails because the handwriting and spelling are ignored as efforts are concentrated on teaching the child to read; an initial attack on the handwriting and spelling would often result in improved reading. Thus, one of the first reasons for emphasizing handwriting is that it helps the child learn to read. In this connection, it is interesting to note that Maria Montessori observed that the very young child writes spontaneously before he reads.

"Write the alphabet" should be a part of every diagnostic testing procedure. The responses and results are often surprising. "All the way through?" – this from an eleven-year-old. "We haven't had *j* in school yet." "I forget how to make *q*." "Which way does *z* go?" In many cases we find that individual letter formation has not been properly learned.

One young adult told me that the worst moment in his school career came in the sixth grade. During the first five grades models of the alphabet had been available in the form of charts posted above the blackboard, enabling him to refresh his memory with surreptitious glances. In the sixth grade the crutch disappeared.

As in all testing, keen observation is essential – of the process as well as of the finished product. We need to watch position and movement of fingers, hand, arm, and paper, as well as direction of letter formation. Certain errors are particularly characteristic of the dyslexic. (See Figure 1.)

In addition, the young child will often print letters such as *f* and *l* beginning at the bottom. Asked to draw a person, he often begins with the feet and works upwards. The more subtle errors in handwriting often linger on after other difficulties have been overcome, and they can be useful, for instance, in deciding why a high school student is failing French and in planning accordingly.

Figure 1

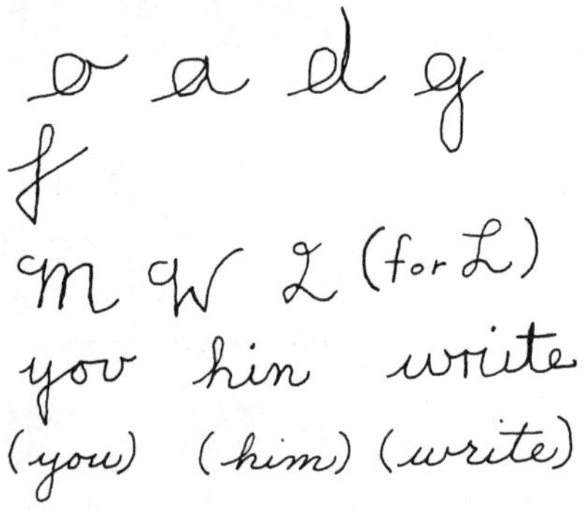

AS A RULE, cursive writing is to be preferred. Opposition to cursive writing is generally founded on the belief that confusion will result from the simultaneous presentation of two alphabets. My experience in teaching in a British school in South Africa has convinced me that this idea is more educational theory than fact. Printing was never taught and the seven-year-olds wrote beautifully, in a style that would be considered good for most fifth graders. Confusion only arises if the children are turned loose to copy the letters without being shown where to begin. Reading is a visual process, writing a kinesthetic one. The two processes do not become confused.

The arguments in favor of cursive writing for dyslexic children are many. In the first place, it seems to help eliminate reversals — the troublesome

b and *d* are less confusing. Secondly, the word is treated as a unit and greater reinforcement is provided for spelling. Then too, with those children who have poor motor control, once they lift the pencil, there is always some doubt as to exactly where it is going to come down. On the other hand, some children with minor brain damage do seem to do better with printing; cursive writing evidently reinforces their tendency to perseverate.

Young children should write with soft pencils or magic markers. Magic markers, unlike chalk, require a firm dragging movement, particularly good for the reinforcement we seek. With older students, the quality of the writing instrument is important — the seventeen-cent ballpoint is rarely adequate as it needs to be held at right angles to the paper in order to function at all. We require good quality ballpoints or pens with medium nibs. Some manufacturers produce very nice pens and pencils with a flared bottom, easy to grip and helpful in preventing students from holding the pen too near the point. Occasionally it is helpful to wrap a couple of rubber bands just below where the index finger and thumb ought to grip.

IN ALL TRAINING or retraining, the first thing to establish is the correct position of the paper, arm, and hand. Paper should be held parallel to the writing arm at about a forty-five degree angle to the table. In some cases, it is helpful to paint parallel "tracks" on the desk or to mark the lines with adhesive tape. For left-handed students, the position is, of course, reversed. The hand not used for writing must be placed firmly, flat on the table on the top of the paper. Only by moving the paper up as he writes is the student able to maintain the correct position. (See Figure 2.) The pencil, held between the index finger and thumb, resting on the third finger, should point towards the shoulder.

Figure 2

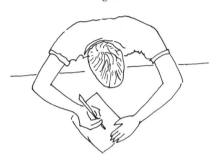

While these preliminaries are being established, it is generally good to start with some sort of scribbling or writing exercise before going on to individual letter formation. The examples in Figure 3 seem helpful, incorporating as they do various writing patterns.

Figure 3

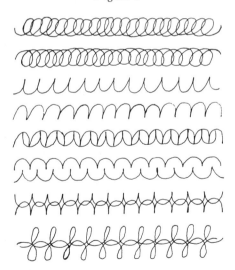

The old-fashioned copy book, still in vogue in many places, owes its popularity to the misconception that writing is a visual process. The child is instructed to look and copy. This method often produces students who glue their eyes to the paper and draw the letters at a painfully slow pace. When they are allowed to write slowly enough, the results are reasonably legible, which fact often proves to the teacher that, "He can write properly when he wants to" — but as soon as he has to write rapidly or spontaneously, or to copy from the chalkboard, the handwriting deteriorates.

TREATING handwriting as a kinesthetic process means that in the initial stages of teaching or of remediation, the student will be instructed to shut his eyes while the teacher moves his hand in the desired pattern. In the case of persistent reversals, the motion may have to be repeated many times before the student is able to reproduce the motion unaided. In order to further reinforce the letter shape, student and teacher name the letter aloud, thereby producing a firm connection between the sound and symbol by using the additional reinforcement, both auditory and kinesthetic.

At first the letters are made large, using the arm muscle, on the air, on the table, on the chalkboard, or on large sheets of newsprint with magic markers. Older children generally obtain equally successful results by writing on ordinary paper with eyes averted or closed. The use of simultaneous oral spelling is continued in all remedial work for a long time, and seems to be the surest method of preventing the slips between brain and hand so characteristic of the dyslexic. Particular attention needs to be paid to the direction of letter formation; for the teacher to observe the finished product is not enough.

Confusion between letters is best handled with some auditory-kinesthetic clue, rather than a visual one, which is as easily reversed as the letter itself. Clues and reminders should always be phrased in the same way. For example, "The *d* starts like *a*"; "The *q* starts like *a* and then goes like *f*"; "The *j* starts like *i* and goes down."

For children having extreme difficulty, separate chants may have to be devised for each letter, along the lines used by physiotherapists working with young children. We teach all letters with an upstroke, either ⌐ or ⌐, depending on the letter. For example, *a, c, d, g, m,* etc., begin thus ⌐ ; and *e, f, h, i,* etc., thus ⌐ . The use of an upstroke helps in the joining of the letters, prevents *d* from looking like *el,* etc., and also helps guard against the tendency to swing into reverse and to make the circles of *a, o, d,* or *g* clockwise. All letters begin in the line and end up in the air thus: *a⌐* .

The rate at which letters are taught and the order in which they are presented varies in individual cases. Sometimes it is best to begin with a small group of easily differentiated letters, as in the Gillingham method;[1] at other times it is best to group letters according to similarity and to learn them in groups. The four bridged letters, *b, o, v,* and *w,* require a great deal of practice in joining with other letters, particularly *r, m,* and *n.*

IF WE ARE working with a child who has already learned to print, allowing him to use printed letters for capitals postpones the task of tackling a second set of letters too soon or before the first is firmly established. Even then, it is best to simplify the capitals by eliminating some of the flourishes. The method shown in Figure 4 usually proves satisfactory.

Figure 4

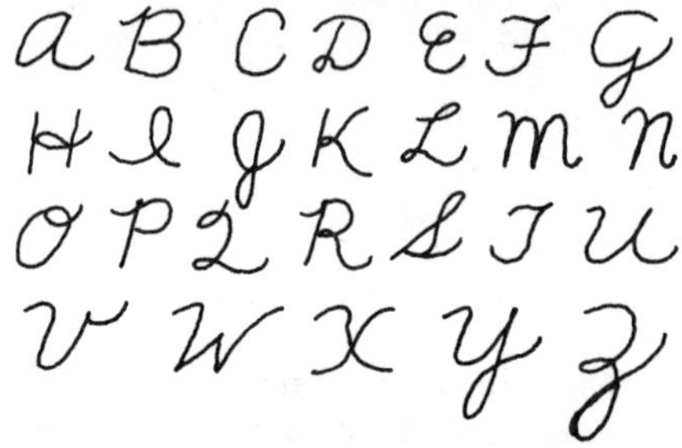

Careful attention must be paid to slant of handwriting. Too often it is assumed that the forward slant is the correct one for everybody. It is safe to say that all left-handed students should write with a back-hand slant. The hooked-wrist position seen so often in the left-handed is inexcusable and, as Miss Gillingham once forcefully expressed it, is always due to the ignorance or laziness of some teacher. If the paper and pencil are held correctly and if the writing slopes backwards from the beginning, the problem never arises in the first place. One excellent first-grade teacher I know used to seat all her left-handed children on one side of the room during writing lessons; placed two models on the chalkboard — those on one side back-hand for the left-handed to copy, and those on the other side forward-slanting for the right-handed.

In training older left-handed children who have already formed the habit of writing incorrectly, the task is somewhat more difficult, but never

---

[1] Anna Gillingham and Bessie Stillman, *Remedial Training for Children with Specific Disability in Reading, Spelling, and Penmanship* (Cambridge, Mass.: Educators Publishing Service, 1960).

impossible. During the retraining process, ideally, no writing should be done outside the remedial lessons, a state admittedly difficult to achieve except during vacations.

It is perhaps less generally realized that many right-handed students also do better with a back-hand slope. In fact, changing the slant is the best way of correcting sprawly, irregular writing. In examining the work of some students, we often note that the letters are slanting in a number of different directions, and that fatigue and haste seem to bring out what may be a natural back-hand slant. Changing the slant often brings a different set of muscles into play — the student has to rely on the large forearm muscle instead of the wrist or the digital muscles, and greater freedom is achieved. There may be psychological benefits in encouraging an adolescent to change the slant of his writing. Certainly the improvement produced time and time again is far greater than would be expected from this simple device.

Figure 5

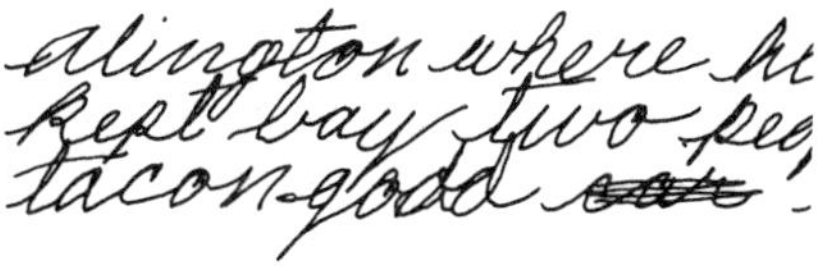

Student A before change of slope.

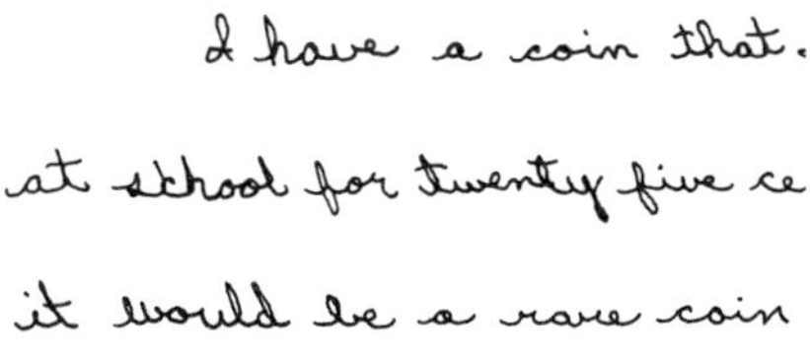

Student A after change of slope.

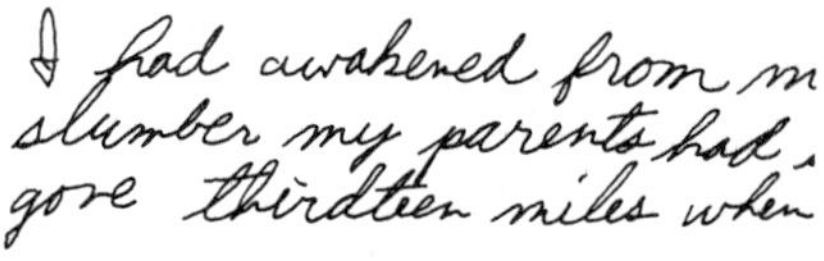

Student B before change of slope.

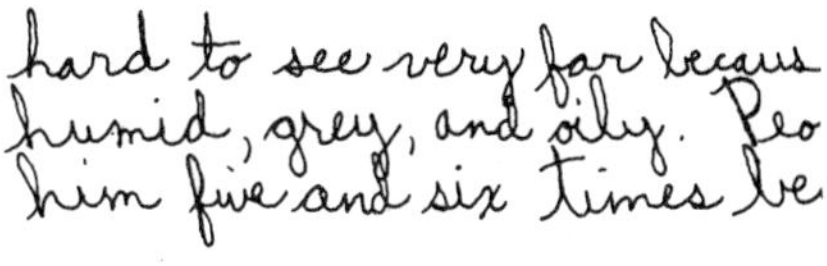

Student B after change of slope.

IN SOME CASES, all our best efforts result in little or no improvement. For such students, the electric typewriter is a boon. Insistence that the typewriter be electric (and perfectly good portable electric typewriters can be purchased now for about $130) is important. There is no need for a student to go to typing school or to work through large numbers of tedious exercises. In the first lesson, we establish the "home keys" and teach the student to write his name in lowercase letters. As he strikes each letter, he names it aloud. In the next two, or occasionally three, lessons we teach the alphabet. Alphabet practice, the student naming each letter aloud, continues for some time. As soon as the alphabet is learned, capitals are added and punctuation is taught. At this stage, there is really no need to teach numerals. The student then begins to type single words, sentences, and paragraphs. Progress is always rapid provided letters are named aloud and eyes are averted from the keyboard.

Typing is useful, not only for the severely agraphic, but for any student who has difficulty in writing and spelling, because it provides one more channel for reinforcement of language.

Some people never learn to spell until they can type. Schools are becoming increasingly flexible in allowing students to use typewriters. Actually, any student above the fourth grade can learn to type in a couple of months on an electric typewriter.

FOR THE DYSLEXIC child, who, while he has one idea in his mind often allows his hand to write something totally different, the teaching of proofreading is important. Older students should be required to proofread all their work. This is a skill that needs to be taught, and which is more difficult than one might think. Once written, the words harden as cement and are as difficult to change. We are all familiar with the omissions, insertions, confusions, substitutions, and reversals of dyslexic children. Proofreading is essential and is preferred to the practice of making a fair copy subsequently. In fact, the making of perfect copies of composition does not work too well with these children. To begin with, they will work too fast the first time round, using the excuse that it is just a rough draft. Then, too, errors will appear in the recopying.

How then, are we to train our students in proofreading? Have him write legibly and, at first, on every other line. If mere reading does not help, ask the student to underline or to circle every word as he checks it, perhaps with red pencil. As the habit of careful scrutiny becomes established, these devices become unnecessary. Later, you can ask him to circle one or two words or set of homonyms which you know he is likely to confuse. Circling or tracing the letters every time they occur helps to eliminate that particular confusion, e.g., *m/n, u/v, b/d*. Probably the very best safeguard against the slips that occur between brain and pen are simultaneous oral spelling and kinesthetic writing, i.e., writing with eyes averted or closed.

The benefits of improved handwriting are many. Handwriting is personal and is very much a part of the student and of the way in which he presents himself to the world. The increased self-confidence engendered by handwriting of which he can be proud is a by-product of no mean value.

Teaching Cursive Writing
to a Perceptually Handicapped Child

Edith Fisher
Christine McMonagle

THE MECHANICAL PROBLEMS of eye-hand coordination and motor control are, for most young children, not easy to overcome when they begin to learn to write. Careful guidance in correct writing habits and much practice are necessary before the child can learn to respond automatically with legible and effortless handwriting.

For the child with perceptual difficulties, this problem is magnified many times. More comprehensive and precise guidance must be given, and more exacting exercises must be devised, in order to help each child over his particular set of hurdles.

Following are some suggestions for helping perceptually handicapped children to achieve in this vitally important and rewarding area of functioning.

The first step is to have the child draw gross circles and diagonals on the blackboard. Thick chalk is useful, particularly when a child holds the writing materials in a spastic-like grip. The child should stand about eighteen inches away from the board and write at eye level. Have him lay the four fingers along the length of the chalk with the thumb on the opposite side. This will allow the use of the side of the point for writing.

When the child begins to write at a desk or table, it is important that he learn the correct sitting position. Have him sit with his hips against the back of the chair and both feet flat on the floor. Both forearms are put on the table, with elbows just off the front edge of the writing surface. Make sure that the child does not have any pressure on the arms, in the knees, or on the feet. This will be difficult and it may help if you suggest to the child that he make his arms and hands feel light and soft as the leg and paw of a friendly kitten.

ANOTHER important point is to teach the child how to align his paper properly. The side of the paper should be parallel with the writing arm. Romalda and Walter Spalding suggest that you tell the child his arm and paper must be like a railroad track.[1] The arm is one track and the edge of the paper is the other. If the child is left-handed, make sure he holds the side of the paper parallel to

[1]
The Writing Road to Reading (New York: William Morrow, 1962.)

79

his writing arm. If the child works at his own desk, a strip of tape placed near the top of the desk at the correct angle will help him to position the top edge of his paper. The slant of the tape will be different for a left-handed child than it is for a right-handed child.

Some children have difficulty in learning to hold a pencil correctly. One method is to put the pencil through the top and bottom of a practice golf ball (the type that has holes all over and is hollow). Have the child place his thumb and index finger around the ball. This forces his fingers into the proper grip.

When the child has learned the correct grip with the golf ball, wind some adhesive tape, *with the sticky side out*, around the pencil at the place where the pencil is to be held. This helps the child to grip the pencil in the correct spot.

THE NEXT STEP is to prepare worksheets for the child. The first sheets should be stencils of the initial writing strokes:

Other strokes may be introduced when the child is ready.

Some of the children may still grip the pencil too tightly and tear the paper by pressing too hard, or they may have difficulty in controlling the pencil enough to stay within lines. To help children with this problem, I bought some craft-sheet copper from a handicraft shop and cut this into desirable sizes. I drew with a stylus and copper tool fairly wide writing lines on the sheet and then placed one row of each of the following exercises on the copper sheet:

If the child veered off from the strokes it was noticeable, since he created faint new lines on the copper.

The use of the copper sheets could be improved upon if it had been possible to have the copper cut or stamped out like a stencil so that the child was unable to tear it. He would then be forced into bringing some of his intact senses into play.

When the child is ready to write on paper, you may find it helpful to take a shirt cardboard and cut out windows (with a razor blade) of one-line, two-line, and three-line height, as shown in the illustration below. The cut out is then placed over the writing paper. First, using the one-line window, teach all of the following letters: *a, c, e, i, m, n, o, r, s, u, v, w,* and *x.* When the child has mastered these letters — with the window to reinforce his height control, and then without the window — follow the same procedure, using the two-line window, for the letters *b, d, h, k, l,* and *t.* Proceed then to the height of three lines, with the letters *f, g, j, p, q,* and *z.*

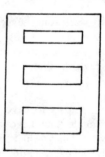

FOR SOME children it may be necessary to establish the starting margin on the paper. This is easily done by running a piece of scotch tape down the margin. If the child cannot stop at the end of the line, a second piece of tape may be run down the right-hand side of the paper. If the child still has difficulty staying within the lines, scotch tape can be used to set up a lesser physical barrier than that provided by the window in the shirt cardboard.

Some children have difficulty discerning which of the three lines is the starting line. If stars are given for good work in your school, the child will be delighted to find a star glued to each starting line as a clue. The star at the beginning of the line will encourage him to even greater effort.

As the child progresses into connected cursive writing, he will be forced into a free flowing motion instead of a stop and start one. Since it is a connected motion, you will notice that the child will be much more relaxed than when he attempts to print. The more relaxed and comfortable the child is, the freer the motion will be and, to bring this full circle, the more relaxed the child will be.

Facile handwriting is an important part of language. The lack of it is a serious and constant handicap. It is well worth the effort to help a child to achieve this skill.

Dear Davey,

Wen we where at camp I swim in the lake very day. The water vas coll but it made me feel good. Ill be home on Wensday

Joey.

Left-Handed Handwriting

Randy Ramos

RIGHT HANDED people, including teachers, sometimes expect left-handed people to write as they do. This is, of course, a fallacy. People are created differently, so there is no reason why they must write in a uniform manner. This paper is based on personal experience. It will serve, I hope, to improve the understanding of right handers, with their "backward" ways. It may also help improve the handwriting of left-handed students who have been trying to write like right handers.

Paper and Hand Positioning.

First of all, the left-handed student must learn to hold his pencil correctly. The pencil must be held with the thumb and the first finger. The second finger bears the weight of the pencil. The back of the hand must be in a straight line with the forearm. If the pencil is not held properly, the hand may smudge the letters. The student should not move his arm while writing, but use his elbow as a pivot point.

Following is a method to help the student position his paper correctly. He should sit at a table or desk and clasp his hands on it, so that his fore-arms are forming a triangle with the edge of the writing surface. He should then place a piece of paper parallel to the writing arm. His paper is now in the proper position.

Pencil Pressure.

If too much pressure is applied to the pencil, the letters will be dark and/or wobbly. One way to test for too much pressure is to turn the student's paper over after he has written on it. If there are small ridges on the back of the paper, too much pressure has been applied.

Wobbly letters indicate a lack of control. With practice and relaxation due to more self-confidence, the letters will smooth out.

Slant.

The slant of left-handed writing should not be the same as for right-handed writing. If the writing is left-handed, the letters should lean slightly to the left. It has been said that a left-handed person writes back-handed. This is not true. Left-handed people should have their letters leaning to the left. The writing is back-handed to people who write with their right hand. The right-handed person writes back-handed too, but this only seems so to the left-handed person.

In rowing, swimming, and gymnastics, the arms of right and left-handed persons have the same movements, but they go in reverse patterns. The right-handed person writes from left to right. The left-handed person writes from left to right. The left-handed person should move in a reversed way, from right to left. We left-handed people compromise and write from left to right, but we slant our letters to the left.

Drawing circles is a good exercise for developing the correct slant.

Left-handed   *circles*

Right-handed   *circles*

Letter Spacing.

If the student is to space letters evenly, he must have good control over each letter. He sometimes watch-

es himself make each stroke, and this slows him down. Sometimes he cannot remember letter forms. If he will look straight forward while writing, he will develop a better sense of feel and will learn to write evenly spaced letters.

IT IS HOPED that the foregoing suggestions, with diligent practice, will help left-handed students to improve their handwriting. It is also hoped that right-handed teachers will be better able to assist their left-handed students in learning to write legibly and easily.

REFERENCES

Gillingham, Anna, and Bessie W. Stillman. *Remedial Training for Children with Specific Disability in Reading, Spelling, and Penmanship.* Cambridge, Mass.: Educators Publishing Service, 1960.

Using the Chalkboard to Overcome Handwriting Difficulties

———————————————

THE DEVELOPMENT of good handwriting is essential to a modern educational curriculum. Penmanship skills must be taught at all levels of the elementary grade school. It must not be left up to the "next year's teacher." A tremendous improvement in handwriting skill is evident when pupils learn to enjoy diagnosing their own handwriting and practicing correct letter formation. This is accomplished by work at the chalkboard.

Using the chalkboard develops a natural body rhythm. There is a free participation of the hand, arm, and fingers in a swinging movement that carries the child along from letter to letter. At the board, the child uses the tactile-kinesthetic method to the best advantage. Many children strengthen their mental imagery through tactile and motor methods rather than through visual and auditory methods. In using this tactile-kinesthetic method on the chalkboard the children are writing at eye level, seeing it, hearing it as they whisper with their work, and feeling it through small muscles in their fingers, hands, and arms. In spelling we write through kinesthetic memory, and in reading this method helps the left-to-right movement of the eyes.

Visualization is a factor of prime importance in learning to write legibly. The child must develop the skill to see in detail the image of the letter or the word. He must also have a mental image of the movements which are necessary in forming letters and words. Examples on the chalkboard are large enough for the young child to see the details of form. They are directly above or adjacent to the child's line of writing. Having the letters enlarged by the teacher and the student aids visualization. The child is really looking at and seeing the letter forms. This makes possible more effective comparison with his own writing. For example, he notes that letters should start at the top and pull down toward the center of the body.

Children should have a chalkboard available to them from an early age. We should encourage scribbling and drawing just for fun. We lead the child from the simple to the more complex. The various strokes are shown as the child needs them. Combinations of letters are practiced, then words (chalkboard writing helps guide the child in the correct sequence of letters here), then sentences. Writing

85

on the chalkboard utilizes the child's arm movements instead of the finger movements of paper writing. Hand-painting and easel painting use and train large muscles also. There needs to be more large-muscle activity as the coordination of smaller muscles of the hands and fingers do not mature as early as the coordination of the larger arm muscles. A child makes large strokes and marks better than smaller ones. This is why we always use and teach the upper-case letters of the alphabet first. Using a piece of chalk — the better for children because of its larger diameter — the child does his work, either copying from the teacher's example or from previous work. His efforts are emphasized and enlarged on the chalkboard.

IN OUR SCHOOL, which has children from preschool through sixth grade in the same room, all ages are writing on their own level, with the younger ages looking forward to becoming as proficient as the older ones, and the older youngsters willingly showing a younger child the correct way to "make a letter" or to spell a word. To quote Mr. Frank Laubach, "Each one teach one" is an acceptable, proper, and effective procedure.

Writing periods are sufficiently flexible to permit individuality in teacher guidance. The program provides definiteness, sureness, and uniformity of purpose. We give due consideration to the individual differences and needs of each child and emphasize correct form and practice habits on the chalkboard. Analysis of letter forms and other study helps are given to the child as he has need of them.

Letters are introduced and practiced in separate examples. This is meaningful to the child as he wants to correct the execution of letters that fall short of being acceptable. Under the teacher's guidance there is given a pattern of repetition of words and letters that gives sufficient practice to develop the skill that is desirable to each growth level.

There is a readiness for cursive writing the same as there is for reading. Research has shown that most of the children are ready to make the transfer from manuscript to cursive writing some time from the latter part of second grade to the beginning of the third grade. Authorities agree that readiness to make the transition from manuscript to cursive writing varies with individual children. Some studies indicate that the majority of children are better equipped to cope with cursive writing without physical or emotional strain after they have entered the third year of school. I have noticed when a child of age four to seven asks for help in cursive writing he is able to cope with it physically and emotionally if reinforced with chalkboard work. With this young child, it takes very little to satisfy social and parental pressure. The parental pressure lessens when these children write just a few things. Their first and last names, address, and city usually suffice. With this pressure relieved, the child is free to evaluate and improve his manuscript in grades one and two.

IF A CHILD is to master the skills necessary in handwriting to a degree that assures legibility and a fair rate of speed, he must engage in systematic and sustained practice and drill at regular intervals. *Drill* need not be a bad word. It can be something to which the child looks forward — awaiting his turn eagerly. We notice that the children's span of attention is comparatively long when working on the chalkboard. Eyes and hands seem not to tire as easily as they do while working on paper and the flat desk top. The child practices on the handwriting skill which he needs, both in school and out of school. Each child knows that this skill is useful and so he realizes that all practice is meaningful.

Drill in writing is a tool and has no value unless it is applied effectively. The children are eager to practice on the chalkboard. They use the chalkboard at other periods. At recess times they are seen helping each other or practicing alone. Their practice is related to all areas in their experience. Some of these areas cover art, health, literature, numbers, phonics, play, reading, safety, science, social studies, and spelling — even labeling in their map making. These are in addition to actual writing situations such as letter writing, reports, announcements, outlining, directions, word study, poetry, and song writing.

The correct pedagogical sequence of going from the simple to the more difficult is being done naturally with the child's own innate ability as his teacher. This natural desire of every child to learn to write well is kept on a high level with activities on the chalkboard. When writing is poor, pupils are hampered in word recognition, pronunciation, and meaning. Mal-

formed letters are a common problem in spelling. In composition, the flow of ideas and the expression of thought are slowed down by poor writing. We all need to set good examples in our own handwriting. We try to lead the child to discover that he writes to be read, and when his writing is legible he is happy and proud of his efforts.

A CHILD is thrilled when he expresses himself in handwriting. Although he needs help in learning concentration and coordination, when good handwriting becomes natural to him he gains emotional security. Learning to write, for the child, is fun — fun in the sense of personal achievement and fun in entertaining his friends and in showing the right way to a child who cannot do a certain letter or word as well as he. The children also realize that there is a purpose and a need for developing good handwriting skills and habits. Each child uses self-evaluation. This is a constant challenge. He is prompted to look for his errors, to engage in independent practice to correct them, and is encouraged to do his best writing at all times.

Interest, purpose, and need — these are motivations that stimulate the child to achieve. They can be sustained and reinforced by daily work on the chalkboard.

The story was about
a boy and his dog.
The dog wanted to
take a walk in the
woods. Bill knew that
the woods were not
safe but Ruff went
anyway. The story ends
when Ruff chases the
bear away.

Mike

Aspects of Visual Development
that Relate to Handwriting

THE PURPOSE OF THIS paper will be to relate, from an optometric point of view, handwriting to child development. These are some of the considerations that optometrists must make when relating the development of handwriting to visual function. Handwriting will be discussed from the point of view of 1. the development of purposeful fine motor control, and, 2. a tool for symbolic encoding.

Studies in child development indicate that the newborn is capable of moving in response to certain stimuli. Most early movement appears to be triggered off by reflex action. For example, breathing and suckling activity seem to be established on a reflex basis. When the feet are caused to be moved by tickling, or some other stimulation, the movement is often accompanied by movement of the arms. This is known as mass action. An infant will turn his head toward the light. This also appears to be a reflex action.[1] Similarly, the aligning of the head in relation to sound also seems to be a reflex action to balance out the energy difference between the neural inputs from the ear.[2] Seemingly, most reflexes are designed to somehow equalize or balance energy differences within the system and hence maintain homeostasis.

From this beginning, the infant learns discrete movement patterns. He learns to move his eyes without necessarily moving his head and shoulders. He learns to coordinate movements of locomotion. He learns to develop a system that is somewhat self-sustaining. To this end, he has made large strides by the time he is eighteen months of age. The system that is developed for coordination and sustaining activities is developed within the organism and the space about. Arnold Gesell implies that by eighteen months, children have discovered that they can cause things to happen about them in space.[3] Often they move

---

[1] The retina is divided into four quadrants by the distribution of nerve fibers in the optic nerve. The vertical separation is caused by the chiasmic decussation. The horizontal line is known as the horizontal raphe. When the energy is equalized in these four quadrants by reposturing of the eye, the eye will be aligned on the light source.

[2] This can be explained from the point of view of both energy difference and phase difference.

[3] Arnold Gesell, *The First Five Years of Life* (New York: Harper and Brothers, Inc., 1940) 33; *Vision, Its Development in the Infant and Child* (New York: Paul Hoeber, 1940) 108

around in their domain just causing things to happen. They push buttons, drop dishes, throw toys, and the like. Seemingly, awareness that they can cause things to happen is not accompanied simultaneously by an awareness of the consequences of the happening. They are interested in the moment, the here and now. Anticipation of the consequences does not seem to occur until later. Many people in child development think of eighteen months of age as the dividing age between infancy and preschool. This would seem appropriate in view of the preceding observations.

From the point of view of handwriting, this preceding development is important. By the age of twelve months, children learn not only to be able to grasp a cube, but also to release the cube as they desire.[4] By eighteen months old, this skill has been extended so that they can often build a vertical tower of three blocks. The very ability to build a tower, however, presupposes that the children look at a tower someone else had constructed and then make one like it. In other words, they must have some model, or idea, developed in their mind of that which they wish to reproduce. Their movements then become purposeful in reproducing this model.

Significant also from the point of view of child development is that the ability to draw a vertical line lags the ability to construct the vertical tower. Most children are able to make purposeful circular and vertical strokes by twenty-four months of age holding the pencil by a Palmer grasp. Here again, it presupposes that the child have some model or representation in his mind that he wishes to reproduce. This will make the difference between a random scribble and a directed line.

By three years old, the child has achieved the ability to make a horizontal line. Diagonal lines follow. From these, children are able to make pictures, and the like.

IN GENERAL, a child first practices the use of pencil and paper through drawing pictures. Later, he learns to form letters. It would seem to be no accident that the earliest known writing of our present civilization is picture writing. Gradually, the pictures were abbreviated into letters. Letters were ultimately developed as a simplification and clarification of the old picture writing technique.

The typical order necessary for the development of suitable handwriting would be: 1. the ability for purposeful fine motor control, and, 2. the discovery of the value of handwriting to encode speech — "Written matter is just talk wrote down."[5] Many children have been introduced to handwriting by learning first to write their name. Sylvia Ashton-Warner introduced children to reading and writing by asking each child to suggest a word he would like to learn that day. No matter how children are introduced to letters, two variables are always present: purposeful fine motor control and symbolization.[6]

---

[4]*Op. Cit.* (1949) 102

[5]Harold E. Brown, *This Is the Way to Study* (New York: Lippincott Co., 1955)

[6]Sylvia Ashton-Warner, *Teacher* (New York: Simon and Schuster, 1963)

The development of goal-seeking, self-directing, and self-correcting fine motor response systems has already been described. Such development generally proceeds from a reflex system that initiates movement, through a period known as mass action, to coordinate gross motor and ultimately fine motor control. It appears to be possible to skip some gross motor development and still have fine motor control. It is possible to be basically awkward in gross motor movements and yet have small handwriting with the letters well formed and rhythmically produced. Often individuals who write this way show good control of the wrist, hand, and fingers but tend to minimize the use of the arm in the handwriting act. They tend to hold their pencil tightly and close to the end. They lean over the task so that their eyes are very close to the paper. It is not unusual for them to develop myopia or nearsightedness.[7]

It is also possible to develop handwriting patterns when gross motor control seems adequate but fine motor control less than adequate. Generally, this type of writing is large and sprawley with the letter formations inconsistent with size. When writing on unlined paper, they generally write up hill or down hill. On lined paper, the letters do not consistently sit on the line. The development of sufficient degrees of freedom in the system to allow smooth and rhythmic formation of the letters comes with practice. It is difficult to adequately express the importance of this phase. On the surface, it would seem that all that is required would be repetitive practice. Seemingly, if one performs a particular action over and over again, he should become automatic and proficient in that act. Yet, this is not always the case. One can also practice in error and become quite good at it. The development of severe limitations may result. For example, one can learn to type using two fingers and become quite proficient. However, a good two finger typist is limited in learning to become a good ten finger typist. Yet, a good ten finger typist can out perform the best of the two finger typists in a varied cross section of typing work. Practice should be more than repetition. Practice should also include a notion of purpose. The purpose or goal may be a visual and kinesthetic pattern that the student desires to create. Later, the goal may be such things as symbolization of a thought, a bit of prose, or encoding a concept of universal unity.

W HAT ARE SOME of the factors involved with developing adequate degrees of freedom in handwriting? Freedom demands the ability of coordinate movement. (Robert Frost says that freedom is the ability to move easy in harness.) Coordinate movement requires a balanced starting point from which to begin the movement. To this end, free handwriting movement should start with appropriate writing posture. The body should be in balance with gravity and the task. To achieve this, it is best to start with the desk appropriately adjusted to the size of the child. Adjustment of the chair height may be considered correct when a child can sit at his desk with both feet flat on the floor, his knees making a right angle bend. The desk should be adjusted to allow the forearm to rest on the edge of the desk while the child is sitting in the above posture and leaning slightly forward. In this posture, the spine of the child should be a smooth curve. The arc of the low back will be minimized. (Contrast this with the stiff "military" posture that once was advocated.)

----

[7]See Dr. Kahn's article in this book.

From the point of view of handwriting, it is ideal to have the desk top tilted at a twenty degree angle from the horizontal rather than be flat.[8] Often this is not possible. To determine the ideal posture for writing on a flat surface, one must first determine the preferred hand and the preferred eye of the student. The preferred hand may be determined by observing which hand is used for holding the pencil when writing.

The eye preference of the child may be determined by standing approximately ten feet in front of the child and having the child extend his preferred arm and point to your nose. Note his sighting eye. This may be considered to be his preferred eye by this test. Another method is to give the child a paper mailing tube about one inch in diameter and ask the child to look through the tube as if it were a telescope. Observe which eye the child uses to look through the tube. This may be considered his preferred eye. [9]

FROM THE DEVELOPMENTAL point of view, many optometrists favor the learning of cursive writing before printing. Historically, the early teaching of printing has come into vogue to theoretically ease the transition between the written letter and the printed page. From empirical observations printing seems to encourage concentration of attention on single letters as individual entities and thus develops a tendency to segment or to work in smaller or more weakly-linked thought units. The learned rhythmic flow of hand movement, especially when taught by the Palmer method seemed to enhance development of fine motor control. Further, it would seem to provide a foundation for flow from letter to letter in rhythmic sequence and ultimately to the development of rhythmic patterns of thinking.

Whether or not the Palmer method enhances future legibility of handwriting is not the issue here. Empirically, it would seem that the teaching of cursive writing before printing would enhance programs of thinking readiness.

Margaret Smith and Karl Smith prepared an experiment whereby a subject was asked to write.[10] He did not view his own handwriting directly as he wrote, but rather saw it on a television screen before him. Adaptation to this situation was not difficult for the subject. This arrangement allowed for varying a variety of situations. In one situation, the size of the letters viewed on the screen was electronically enlarged. The mismatch between the kinesthetic pattern of writing and the larger visual feedback of the viewed image did not significantly disturb the handwriting performance of the subject. The same was true when the viewed letters were made smaller on the television screen.

---

[8]Since other papers in this collection discuss proper posture, the reader is referred to them.

[9]Darell Boyd Harmon, *Coordinated Classroom* (Published by the author, 1949); *Dynamic Theory of Vision* (Published by the author, Austin, Texas, 1949); *Eye Preference, Certain Body Mechanics and Visual Problems* (Published by the author, Austin, Texas, 1963); "A Preliminary Report on a Study of Eye Preference, Certain Body Mechanics and Visual Problems," *Learning Disorders*, Vol. 2, J. Hellmuth (ed.) (Seattle, Washington, Special Child Publications, 1969).

[10]Karl U. Smith and Margaret Faltz Smith, *Cybernetic Principles of Learning and Education Design* (New York: Holt, Rinehart and Winston, 1966).

In the second situation, the subject was asked to enlarge his own handwriting. When the subject was asked to vary the size of his handwriting, significant disturbances were recorded. The same was observed when the subject was asked to miniaturize his handwriting.

This observation would support the notion that efficient handwriting flows and becomes automatic.

There is evidence to indicate that readiness needs of young school children include an ability known as automatization.[11] This allows learned movement patterns to eventually become automatic. Formerly this development has been taken for granted. The evidence suggests it can be trained as a skill. It would seem that the Palmer method of cursive handwriting would allow itself more to this purpose than would printing.

Another facet related to handwriting would include grasping the writing utensil. Most children learn to write first with a crayon or a pencil. Many children grasp the pencil in a tight manner. The index finger will develop a concave curve. Often the fingernail is white where the circulation to the fingertip has been reduced because of the pressure of the writing grasp. Along with the pencil or crayon such a grasp is also possible with a ball point pen. Ball point pens will allow one to bear down hard on the paper. A suggestion for teaching the children to hold the pencil or pen lightly would be to have them use a type of fountain pen. With a fountain pen, the ink flows freely with very little pressure. Indeed, when too much pressure is exerted, the pen point will bend. It may even become damaged.

Further, it is important that the child grasp the writing utensil lightly between the tips of the thumb and middle finger with the tip of the index finger on top of the implement. This allows for finger-tip control of the writing utensil and thus allows for greater sensitivity and development of fine motor control. Indeed, a strong indication of the lack of fine motor control is the holding of the pencil by the sides of the fingers rather than by the fingertips.

It might be asked why the handwriting of many creative individuals appears to be illegible. There are probably many reasons for this. One of these would include the observation that creative people are often biased in terms of a particular point of view, or talent. As such, it would be natural that they reflect these biases in all muscle tensions of their body. This in turn would affect all motor outputs including handwriting.

Another explanation might be suggested by the observation that many of the proper writing habits that have been learned in the early grades tend to change and vary as the individual begins to use writing as a tool for symbolizing or encoding verbal language. It would seem that "the thought becomes the thing" rather than the motor encoding process. As such, less attention is directed to legible letter formation, and the like. The writer only requires enough of a clue from the encoding process to be able to reintegrate the thought. He does not require the redundancy of legible handwriting. Consequently, handwriting suffers.

---

[11]David Whiting, Melvyn Schnall, and Charles Drake, *Automatization in Dyslexic and Normal Children* (Wellesley, Mass.: Reading Research Institute, 1968)

A DISCOURSE ON THE developmental aspects of handwriting should not end without at least attempting to relate the development of handwriting to the development of specific types of information processing in children. It is commonly accepted that there are at least three fundamental modes of learning: the kinesthetic mode, the auditory mode, and the visual mode. It seems that one must develop an integration of at least two modes before they operate effectively. When one is operating primarily through but one mode, severe learning disabilities ensue and handwriting will be affected. This seems particularly true with children operating primarily through the kinesthetic and the kinesthetic-auditory mode.

Behaviorally, the motor development of kinesthetic children is slow. They may not turn over in their cribs until nine months old, they may not have any desire to crawl, and attempts to encourage crawling may meet with further resistance to crawl.

When they are raised in a home where they are loved and "smushed," they are generally happy babies. They thrive on love, being cuddled, and the like. Even as preschool children, they seem to crave physical contact in the form of hugs and squeezes from their parents. They smile a lot, eat, and sleep well. They are the picture of contentment. They lie there happily, but do not move. Perhaps there is no need to move.[12]

When they are raised in an environment where they did not receive the physical contact and affection they crave, they are apt to be insecure, prone to nightmares, cry more frequently, develop spastic movements, and the like.

Characteristically, these children do not learn through spankings. They are shocked and confused by spankings. The confusion seems to limit learning. However, they respond less well to the "progressive school of thought"; they need direction. As with all children they seem to respond most fully to *consistent* loving discipline.

Paradoxically, these children appear to have their kinesthetic system as one of their primary modes of learning. Some may like to listen to music and rock in their chairs indicating an associated auditory mode. Others may wish to sit and observe others indicating an associated visual mode.

It seems paradoxical because one might believe that because the kinesthetic system plays a major role in manipulation of the environment and hence the development of integrated learning patterns within all sensory modes, that someone with a dominance of kinesthetic processing should be an expert manipulator. From empirical observation, the converse seems to be more prevalent. For example, many children who appear kinesthetically dominant appear awkward in their motor patterns. They do like to touch items in space and explore through touch. They enjoy body contact. However, often they are clumsy and succeed in breaking and destroying the item. When the item does not work to

---

[12]My estimate is that these children would include about 5 percent of my patient population. In my mind, these are the only groups of children who would qualify for the category of dyslexic contrasted with the many developmental problems who are presently placed under the classification of dyslexic.

their satisfaction, they are apt to become impatient or bored, both of these being avoidance responses.

Seemingly, the problem with the kinesthetic individual is that he does not "look before he leaps," but tends rather to plunge blindly into the situation. Consequently, the kinesthetic individual tends to lack self-direction.

The kinesthetic system is a powerful system. It has at least three main areas of function: 1. the proprioceptive area or awareness of body parts, 2. the awareness and memory of movement of the body parts, and 3. the association of various moods and emotions that are related to movement of body parts.

It has been established by Richard Held and his associates that effective learning or relearning requires self-direction and self-correction.[13] Only then can appropriate feedback loops be developed for recall and extrapolation of experience. Needless to say, the visual system is of major importance in directing the action of the system. Indeed, Gesell observes that "ocular apprehension precedes manual prehension" at four weeks.[14] The typical child begins to "look before he leaps" at about twenty months of age.[15]

Being kinesthetically dominant, it is conceivable that these children do not learn to appreciate the role of visual or auditory information. As such, they lack the pace-setting system for establishing goals. Consequently, they tend to become ensconced in their own self-awareness and have no reason or purpose to learn to move and develop into gross and fine motor movement patterns. The information from the goal-seeking systems of vision and/or audition is not integrated with the motor systems of the kinesthetic and the system then lacks self-direction and self-correction.

It seems important that the "kinesthetic" child be described in a discussion on handwriting because in general, their fine motor control is lacking and their handwriting is a disaster. Along with handwriting exercises, these children need to learn how to look and listen. They need to learn to appreciate the goal-seeking, anticipatory sense that can evolve through the integration with the visual and auditory modes.

It is not unusual to have handwriting improve with these children through a program of visual training, even when no specific emphasis has been placed on handwriting per se. Yet through a program of visual training, one learns to coordinate the action of the total system in relation to the visual information. The visual system becomes the goal-seeking, pace-setting system which allows for kinesthetic direction and correction of the motor system to achieve results.

---

[13]Richard Held and Alan Hein, "Adaption of Disarranged Hand Eye Coordination Contingent upon Reafferent Stimulation," *Perceptual and Motor Skills*, 8, 1958, 87-90; Richard Held and Jerold Rekosh, "Motor Sensory Feedback and the Geometry of Visual Space," *Science*, 141:3582, 1963; Richard Held, "Plasticity in Sensory-Motor Systems," *Scientific American*, 213:5, 1965; Richard Held, et al, "Altered Teaching Following Adaptation to Optical Displacement of the Hand," *Journal of Experimental Psychology*, 73:1, 1967.

[14]*Ibid.* (1940)

[15]*Ibid.* (1949)

In summary, we have discussed handwriting in terms of child development from an optometric point of view. We have discussed handwriting from the point of view of the development of fine motor control and as a tool for symbolization. We have alluded to handwriting in the process of creating. Finally, we have made some observations of one type of behavior which seems to have particular difficulty in developing fine motor control and hence legible handwriting.

The Developmental Process of Handwriting

Aletha P. Thomas

WRITING, like speech, is a form of communication. Just as speech depends on sound symbols, writing depends on visual symbols. While speech and writing are expressive means of communication, reading is the receptive means of communication.

It is noted that language has three functional categories: inner, receptive, and expressive. Speech must be received and perceived (inner and receptive) before speech as oral language (expressive) is produced. Reading is the result of both adequate oral communication and adequate visual response to printed symbols (perception). Therefore, reading must await spoken language. Further, "Written language is the expressive side of read language," so written language must await both oral and read language. Inadequacies in any one of the three functions can be disruptive of one or more of the other functions of the communication area.

Language also involves three systems: the peripheral nervous system, the central nervous system, and the emotional nervous system. Malfunction or dysfunction in one or more of these three systems can impair language development in an individual.

Impairment of the peripheral nervous system, such as blindness or deafness, interferes with those language processes which are dependent on the involved sensory functions. Impairment of the central nervous system may impede development of one or more of the four types of verbal symbols. Emotional trauma may inhibit one or more of the functions of developmental language.

WRITTEN communication occurs last in language development and therefore is dependent on the completed processes of oral expression (to speak) and symbol reception (to read). To write, the spoken sounds must be reproduced in the read symbols and must have form and meaning. Letter symbol form (writing) and letter arrangement (spelling) must be reproduced first as a visual image or in the "mind's eye" and be available for use (recall).

Visual conceptualization of space and position are necessary to place symbols for legibility. Of course, for writing to be truly communicative, words must be available for transferring and writing thoughts and ideas. Of utmost importance is the *need* or *desire* to produce written communication.

The Role of Vision.

SINCE visual stimuli cannot occur in the blind, writing of letter symbols is generally impossible. This is suggestive of the role that adequate visual stimuli must play for motor direction in handwriting.

The importance of the eye directing the hand to produce the written word can be pointed up by a simple experiment. With the eyes closed, attempt to write a few lines. There appears to be a deluge of learned visual stimuli attempting to move the hand in what the "mind's eye" feels is adequate space, position, and direction. The mind attempts to conjure words and thoughts from a "blind" and frustrated thought process.

The mind's eye is attempting to direct the hand without benefit of the visual assistance which gives physical dimensions for space and position (spatial relationships). Handwriting requires visual monitoring.

Fine motor activities, such as writing, also require adequate ocular balance. Try reading a book while moving it forward and backward through the point of convergence. This somewhat simulates the malfunction of ocular imbalance and might be suggestive of writing under the same condition.

Further experimentation can be tried for simulating malfunctioning visual perception. Write a sentence in manuscript using words containing *w*, *m, d,* and *b.* Write the first word in reverse, the next correctly (forward), write a word with *w* inverted, one with *m* inverted, and another with the *b* and the *d* reversed.

What has been suggested is that for us to attempt the opposite of what we visualize is what occurs with youngsters having visual disorders of varying degrees or kinds. To begin with, these malfunctions impede reading ability and there would appear to be a compounding of difficulties by the demand for production of written expression.

Attempts to press children for paper and pencil activities before there has been adequate growth, development, and eye-hand experimentation perpetuates further "break-down" and invites *more* emotional overlay.

The Need for Readiness.

DEMANDS for handwriting or any activity which necessitates the combined efforts of systems not yet neurologically, emotionally, and physiologically developed can produce unnecessary repercussions for a child.

Written communication is the least necessary tool in the early years of a child's school life, yet this is the most pressed-for and the most demanded skill — even more so than reading.

If we consider neurological growth as developing from the body center outward, the large muscles and their neurological controls must precede the fine muscles and their neurological growth. This represents developmental order. Activities must be allowed which encourage this growth pattern.

Unnecessary blocks result from pushing children into by-passing growth and developmental stages and not allowing them to wait for "readiness."

*Neurological and Visual
Compensations.*

THE LEFT-HANDED child with the "back-handed" writing position and the "fist writer" are familiar examples resulting from demands made on the child before sufficient growth and readiness have taken place.

The child who chooses the left hand for dominance is moving against neurological growth in writing. The position of the paper and pencil require that the left hand move toward the body center. This is a neurological factor.

When paper and pencil are in the "proper" position for writing, the left hand interferes with vision both by its movement and by its covering effect. Many left-handed children develop "claw" or back-handed writing habits to compensate for these interferences. This is a visual factor.

BACK-HANDED writing places the hand and the writing instrument above the line of writing. This demands that the writer curve the wrist, thus placing the hand at a right angle to the forearm and the writing implement parallel to the forearm with its top end pointing away from the writer. The writer now writes parallel to the body, using finger movement only. By further adjustment of the paper to the right-hand position, the writer gains a right-hand slant to the letter form.

The "fist writer," usually left handed, presses the pencil between the first and second knuckle of the forefinger, using the thumb as the point of pressure for holding the instrument. All fingers are doubled into the fist position, which gives the appearance of amputated fingers. This is painful to see and tiring and painful for the writer. This would appear to be indicative of the "splintering-off" which Dr. N. C. Kephart referred to as a neurological factor, it being symptomatic of restricted motor approach.

The fist writer leans heavily on the hand, and movement is limited to thumb and forefinger. This type of writing may be employed in conjunction with either back-handed writing or an upside-down position of the paper.

The left-handed writer who turns the paper upside-down for writing is not seen as often as the "backhander," perhaps, but it offers two escapes. The paper is placed so that the child is writing away from the midline and the hand no longer interferes with the child's vision.

Two points should be emphasized here. Any child showing gross muscle difficulties or displaying deficiencies in activities requiring fine finger movement should not be expected to participate in paper and pencil tasks. The other point to be noted is that once a child has decided on a method for writing, holding the pencil, and positioning of the paper, it is almost impossible to implement any appreciable changes.

Symbol Form Patterns.

IT HAS been my experience that children with deep emotional distress display numerous variations in letter or symbol form. These children have a capacity for producing neat and "correctly" formed symbols and may either do so or they may produce distorted symbols. There can be a lack of consistency with the emotionally disturbed child. Just as distress may be noted by distortions in voice pitch, so also may distress be noted by distortions in written symbols.

The neurologically handicapped child does not display this wide range of ability to distort unless he has motor mobility. However, many of the neurologically involved children have not learned this mobility prior to learning a writing pattern; therefore, their distress is demonstrated in messy papers or in nonproductivity (which is also true of the emotionally disturbed).

This information is of importance only in that it serves to remind the teacher that there are other activities that are far more meaningful to these youngsters than is writing.

The child who reverses and inverts symbols and words in reading will do so as well in writing. There are a number of methods being practiced for assisting the child externally, but unless the internal malfunctions can be corrected, then drawing lines under words, teaching cursive instead of manuscript word production, using colored letters for word beginnings, etc., have little lasting value.

Summary.

THE CHILD who does not read has no great need for writing. In the development of language functions, writing is last and should be allowed to follow the developmental schema. The young child should not be pressed for paper and pencil activities. Ample time for growth should be allowed.

The use of manipulative toys makes no demand on the child to excel and opportunity for such activities should be made. There are wide selections of toys and inexpensive materials available which are meaningful and which offer growth time for children. *The child should learn to use all of his body before he is asked to "splinter off" parts for specializing.*

If we can allow ourselves the luxury of waiting for the child's readiness, a few demands for holding a pencil and positioning the paper are all that will be required for the production of the written word.

Once a child begins meeting the social demands for written productivity, he will insist on continuing no matter how awkward or restricting the act of producing may be.

The child has a lifetime in which to practice writing, so why must we insist that he devote so much of his young life to an activity which is useless to him for childhood functioning.

REFERENCES

Kephart, N. C. *The Slow Learner in the Classroom.* Columbus, Ohio: Charles E. Merrill, 1960.

Myklebust, Helmer R. "Language Disorders in Children," *Exceptional Children*, (January 1956), 163-166.

Handwriting Readiness:
Motor-Coordinative Practices

Geraldine M. Kimmell

———————◆———————

WHAT IS the meaning of the term *readiness?* To some it may convey a state of willingness or eagerness to attend to a task or the promptness with which it is performed. To others it may denote the ease or facility with which a performance is executed. However, the state of readiness that is relevant to the acquisition of learning skills should indicate a state of preparedness — a state of being ready not only to understand the principles of the task prescribed but also of being capable physically to undertake the activity. Early training toward this preparedness — preceding the child's attempt to write — is, therefore, as important to success in undertaking handwriting as is the special training preparatory to undertaking reading.

The coordinative muscular action that is involved in executing any form of handwriting seems to be a voluntary action for most persons, but for many individuals, and in particular for the dyslexic or disgraphic, the effort involved in executing handwriting makes it a serious and frustrating experience. The result of this labored effort is a stilted and nonfluent pattern of symbols. This forced endeavor requires such rigid concentration that extreme fatigue can result. Just to properly grasp a writing instrument poses a real challenge for many children.

When this difficulty is noted in a child, it may be that the finger muscles, particularly the finer ones, have not been fully developed. This condition could be attributed to an insufficiency of manipulative practice in infancy. All small children should experience hour after hour of handling, twisting, grasping, clutching, and squeezing objects in order to develop the finer muscles of the hands and fingers in a natural and gradual way. If this development has not taken place in the stages of early maturation, exercises must be included in a conditioning program as soon as the deficit is detected, so that a normal acquisition of handwriting skills may be assured for the individual.

Among the many effective exercises that have been developed for this purpose, the following ones, which can be performed with the common, everyday objects that are available in most classrooms or homes, have proved helpful for many students.

Exercise I

· Obtain a small rubber ball (approximately two inches in diameter).

· Ask the student to extend his arm with the palm of his hand downward so that he may determine a comfortable height for bouncing the ball and catching it on the rebound. After asking the student to squeeze the ball tightly for a second as he grabs it on the rebound, repeat this action — (1) bounce, (2) catch, and (3) squeeze — counting aloud to help the student to perform the task rhythmically. Work up to repeating the action ten times with each hand.

· Ask the student to alternate the action by bouncing the ball with the *left* hand and catching and squeezing it with the *right* hand.

Exercise II

· Select a given number of paper clips (vary the number according to the interest and adaptability of the student).

· Ask the student to hold a clip in his subdominant (nonwriting) hand and then pick up a second clip with his dominant hand. Instruct him to link the second clip to the first by twisting it between the bent wires in order to make a chain. The student should continue to link each successive clip to the chain until the given number of clips has been used.

· After the student becomes adept in this manipulative phase, introduce a rhythmic procedure with a metronome to see how fluently and efficiently the student can perform the task — without undue frustration.

· If colored paper clips are available the girls may want to wear the chains as necklaces.

Exercise III

· Obtain a pair of wire-spring plastic or wooden clothespins. (The size of the pin and the strength of its spring should be determined by the student's capability (or comfort) in the manipulation of it.

· Ask the student to grasp the pin in his dominant hand. He should place his thumb on the top shaft of the pin, and the index and middle fingers on the lower shaft. Begin the opening-closing procedure slowly, so that when the student applies pressure to open the pin he becomes aware of the movement of the small muscles involved. The pattern of action is (1) open, (2) hold, (3) close.

· Have the student repeat this pattern as many times as he can perform it comfortably. Care must be taken not to overtire the student. Exerting this type of pressure on weak muscles can not only be exhausting but can, in turn, frustrate the individual beyond his physical endurance, thereby defeating the initial purpose of the exercise.

· If the student cannot open the pin by himself — that is, if the spring is too strong to allow him to open the pin completely without his fingers slipping off the shafts — then the instructor should put his hand over the student's and help him apply the necessary amount of pressure. This "helping hand" is also necessary to assist the child in establishing a given rhythmic pattern for fluency. A metronome may be used. Start the action with the indicator on the metronome set at sixty. Increase the speed as the student develops proficiency in the exercise.

Exercise IV

· Assemble a variety of small articles, such as beads, buttons, beans, macaroni pieces, pennies or dimes, or small nuts.

· If, for example, three articles are chosen to be sorted, locate three boxes and label each one with the name of each of the articles. If buttons, pennies, and nuts are chosen, put all of the buttons in the button box and all of the pennies and nuts in their respective boxes. After putting the boxes on the desk in front of the student, ask him to pick up a button and place it in the box that contains the pennies; next, ask him to pick up a nut and place it in the box that holds buttons; and last, ask him to pick up a penny and place it in the box that contains the nuts. Continue in this manner until all of the buttons are in the penny box, all of the nuts are in the button box, and all of the pennies are in the nut box.

· Alternate or vary this procedure in any way that will make it interesting for the student. The student may close his eyes while doing the exercise, or do it with the boxes behind him — if the teacher feels that more complexity is essential.

Exercise V

· After securing a set of jacks and a small rubber ball, ask the student to practice tossing the ball and catching it before he starts to play the game, particularly if he has not played it before. If he tries to play the game before he can control this action successfully he will give up too soon. The action of grabbing the jacks is just as important in strengthening the hand muscles as is the squeezing of the ball.

Exercise VI

· Obtain a typewriter — a primary keyboard, if possible. Ask the student to strike the keys with a firm pecking action so that clear impressions result. Allow sufficient time for the student to locate the correct letter or number that is dictated in order to assure as little frustration as possible.

· Alphabetical and numerical sequences, specific words from the student's basic vocabulary, or simple sentences are suggestions for dictation.

· The student should continue this exercise until a substantial gain in rhythmic fluency has been attained. (No attempt to teach professional typing is intended.)

Exercise VII

· After thirty-six thumb tacks and a yardstick are placed before the student, ask him to press each tack firmly into the yardstick at one-inch intervals. Next, ask the student to pull out each tack and again press it firmly into the yardstick at the one-half-inch markings. Repeat this pattern several times, or in accordance with the student's endurance.

· A metronome can be used to establish fluent actions.

AFTER the student has practiced these exercises and has made a conscious effort toward their execution, he will have gained a proficiency in muscular coordination, which will afford him a comfortable physical performance during the act of handwriting. He will take pride in his achievement, and he will be happier because of his physical well-being.

ThE school is cool. BuT whEn
I cAmE I wAs A Fool
BuT I FElT liKE I nEvEr CAmE
To School
JusT liKE A cool Fool
I nEvEr lEArnEd And
I nEvEr lisTEnEd ThaTs
how I goT inTo This
condiTion
Now I'M doing bETTEr
by My own AdMission

by DAViD
4th gradE

Big Chalkboards For Big Movements

Harold B. Helms

A TOOL that we have found indispensable at our clinic in San Rafael, California, for helping children who have poor handwriting, is the regular classroom chalkboard — but we turn it on its side. Commercial chalkboards are available usually in 4′ x 6′, 4′ x 8′, and 4′ x 12′ sizes. Homemade varieties are possible by using masonite or other smooth boards and applying chalkboard paint (usually available from the local hardware store) to the surface. The finished product, painted while it is flat, and sometimes needing two coats of paint, may not have the same smooth surface as its commercial counterpart, but it does the job quite well. Two of these boards (4′ x 6′ or 4′ x 8′, depending on the size of the children and the height of the room) can be placed side-by-side and easily mounted to the wall with a minimum of nails, which will give eight linear feet of surface space. "The point at which the two boards meet will create a slight bump as the child writes, but for the exercises described here, this is not critical. If it is disturbing to the child, then use just one surface.)

The purpose of the two high boards, placed side-by-side, is to develop a total body awareness to the kinesthesis of handwriting.

Over the years, in working with children with minimum to severe learning problems, we have found that a great many do not have a well-integrated concept of their own body and its position in space. Quite often the students are tight and rigid, and they move and write in these ways. Other children are loose and disorganized, and they, in turn, move and write in these ways. Their poor posture and coordination is reflected in the slant and formation of the letters and words they write.

When we started to use the big chalkboards, we asked the children to bend from the waist and to reach to the very bottom of the chalkboard, which rested on the floor. We found that a large number had difficulty in doing this — they tightened their fists, and they kept their heads upright.

In order to overcome these difficulties, and to build in ease and fluidity of movement, we had these children practice just bending from the waist. Weighted objects, such as sandbags held in the hands, helped to give the feeling of weight to the arms and

105

helped to reinforce the concepts of up and down — so necessary to writing letters and words. We even found that rolling on a thick carpet helped to loosen tight, rigid bodies and that general coordination improved.

The use of the tall chalkboards was introduced when the child could comfortably bend from the waist. We asked each child to verbalize his movements as he wrote each letter. For example, if the child was writing the letter *h*, he bent so that the hand holding the chalk was at the very bottom of the chalkboard. As he moved up, he would say "up" (and it is important that he reach as high as he can). As the child went back down to the floor, he would say "down," and as he made the hoop he would say "and around" and then "back down."

The child ends up with an *h* that is four feet wide and possibly five to six feet high. He has *felt* the letter with his entire body and has actually experienced a kinesthetic awareness of the shape of the letter. By repeating the activity he builds-in a fuller integration of the form. We have found that it is not necessary, in all cases, to write all letters of the alphabet this way. The children seem to establish movement generalizations. Therefore, they can often repeat the same letter if they wish, or do others. Of course, the program for each child will differ, and the teacher or therapist will have to become an astute judge as she observes the child's reactions and responses, both at this specific task, and in the conventional forms of handwriting. As, however, the child develops proficiency, he can write full words, bending over and stretching high, reaching from left to right, covering the full eight feet.

This approach has helped a large number of children to get the *feel* of letters. We have found that through the use of this technique, the demands of paper-and-pencil tasks — which were so often desperately frustrating — became fluent and comfortable. The child, through experiences such as these is far better equipped to use handwriting as another tool to express himself, efficiently and effectively.

Should Your Child Write with the Left Hand?

A Note for Parents

Dean Trembly

———————————◆———————————

W HAT ARE the chances that your baby will be left handed? Well, that depends partly on the person you have chosen to marry. And, of course, it depends partly on you. What are the chances that all of your children will be southpaws? The answers are the same.

If you happen to be a right-eyed person (the surest indicator being the eye used in peeking through a knot hole in a board fence) and if you pick a right-eyed mate, all of your children will be right-eyed and most likely right-handed. If you are left-eyed and marry a right-eyed person, about one-fourth of your children will be left eyed. But if both you and your mate are left-eyed, all of your children will be left-eyed and you will have a family of southpaws, provided neither imitation nor intimidation interferes.

Such predictions are possible because of the same Mendelian law of inheritance that allows two genuine blonds who marry to predict that all of their children will be blonds. Left-sidedness, as well as blond hair, appears to be a recessive genetic trait, always reproduced in the child when both parents have the trait.

However, an exception to the rule is found in each pair of identical twins. Cell division, which produces identical twins, causes one twin to be the opposite of the other in eye dominance. Exceptions to the genetic rule of recessives also may occur in cases where only one twin survives the embryonic stage.

How to Determine Sidedness in an Infant

Y OU MAY HAVE observed in new-born infants a posture resembling a fencing attitude; head to one side with the arm on the same side extended and the arm on the other side bent toward the shoulder. Each infant, even the premature seven-month one, seems to prefer such a one-sided position whether lying face up or down. In the Clinic of Child Development at Yale University, Dr. Arnold Gesell found that this tonic-neck-reflex posture, in which the infant faces and extends his hand to either the right or left, is the first sign of inborn sidedness. You may notice also on this dominant side a greater amount of activity in the hand, wrist, fingers, foot, ankle, and toes.

After the first twelve weeks, the process of development begins to involve more diverse movements. You will begin to notice your baby facing both ways and moving his hands more equally. Although the general trend from birth to maturity is toward a preferred use of the muscles of one side of the body, evidence of transfers and retransfers of sidedness during the three to twenty-four month period is presented by both Dr. Gesell and others. He calls this shuttling back and forth "Reciprocal Interweaving." It is part of the growth process which brings into working balance the two sides of the human organism.

You probably will notice several shifts of hand preference during this phase of growth. Do not be alarmed. This is normal. You will find it difficult to remain neutral but it is very important that you make no final decision at this time as to which hand your baby should use. One mother noticed that her seven month old son had started to use his left hand. Desiring to be a progressive mother and to avoid any ill effects of enforced right-handedness, she immediately began training him to be left handed. He grew up writing and eating with his left hand, but using his right hand in all other activities. Not until the age of fourteen when an eye dominance test showed him to be right eyed, did the mother realize that she had made her decision at too early an age on insufficient evidence.

If you have had a chance to determine your child's sidedness immediately after birth, you will be interested in his final preference after the completion of the reciprocal interweaving process. The two should agree. If they do not, or if your child is already past his first twelve weeks when you read this, you should wait until he is about two years old before deciding which is the correct hand to use. In making this decision, you are actually deciding on his writing hand, although his writing comes later.

How to Determine Sidedness — 24 Months to 5 Years

NATURAL SIDEDNESS seems to be firmly established by the age of 24 to 30 months. From this age onward the surest indication of sidedness is the use of the dominant eye in sighting. Cut a hole about the size of a quarter in a large piece of cardboard and teach your child to play peek-a-boo through the hole. You can be fairly certain of his eye dominance if he consistently uses the same eye and if you are positive that he is not blind in the other eye. If he uses first one eye and then the other, you should defer judgment until a replaying of the game at monthly intervals produces consistent results. If you are still not sure which is the preferred sighting eye, begin to watch which hand he uses in untrained activities. When he hits something, which hand does he use? How does he throw, pick up an object, or play games? Preference of the left hand after the age of 24 months in small, ordinarily unnoticed behavior is a good clue. Not until a definite preference is reached are you justified in training him to use the hand corresponding to the dominant eye.

Imitation Can Work Either Way

ACTUAL TRAINING is more often needed in families where the left-eyed baby is surrounded by friendly right-handed people, whom he tends to imitate, or where the right-eyed baby is being raised by a left-handed mother. The story of one man, a vice-president of a cotton oil mill near Fort Worth, illustrates this danger. He was right eyed but left handed, a rare combination. He said that both of his parents were right handed and he expressed wonder at his being left handed. It was suggested that he ascertain the eye dominance of his parents when he next visited them, and that he ask them of his childhood associations. He found that both parents were indeed right eyed, as well as right handed, but that in his infancy, at which time the family lived in Virginia, much of his care had been entrusted to a nurse who was left handed.

A recent survey of handedness in the schools of one city found that almost half of the children in two first grade rooms of a parochial school were learning to write with their left hands, an incidence far in excess of the twelve percent found elsewhere. Further investigation revealed that both of the teachers involved were left handed and were unaware that so many of their students were copying their handedness in writing.

How to Determine Eye Dominance — 5 Years and Up

As the child matures, the preferred eye in sighting remains the most reliable indication of natural sidedness. You may observe in some children that the sighting eye is the weaker of the two. This is not uncommon, for there is no relation between eye strength and eye dominance.

For adults, and for children who have outgrown the age of peek-a-boo, you may use a card about nine by twelve inches with a hole in the center the size of a dime. On a second card, or on a piece of paper, draw a pair of crossed lines, each line running diagonally from one corner of the paper to the opposite corner. The place where the two lines cross will be the sighting point.

Instructions for Sighting

1. Keep both eyes open. Hold the card having the hole with both hands, arms extended and lowered.

2. Look across the room at the card having the crossed line.

3. Keep looking (both eyes open) at the point where the lines cross and, still holding your card at arm's length, raise your card until you can see the cross through the hole.

4. Repeat this three times. Keep both eyes open.

5. After you have raised the card for the third time, keep looking at the cross through the hole. Without losing sight of the cross, slowly pull the card toward your face until it touches your nose. Hold it there.

6. Decide which eye is looking through the hole by closing first one eye and then the other.

7. The eye looking through the hole is your dominant eye.

8. Repeat several times.

9. Close the eye which was used in sighting. Keep it closed. Using the other eye, sight through the hole at the cross. This is done to learn if your other eye can see, for only if both eyes can see is the sighting test a true indicator of inherent sidedness.

Why Write with Your Left Hand?

"In this predominantly right-handed world why should anyone with good sense deliberately train his child to write with the left hand?" some parents ask. This is a practical question. Stated in more general terms the question might be, "Why should the left-eyed quarter of the population be left handed?" The companion question, "Why should the right-eyed three quarters of the population be right handed?" also needs to be answered.

Neurologists have described the relation of sidedness to the two hemispheres of the brain. A specific nerve area in one hemisphere has its counterpart in the other. The corresponding areas function in unison in receiving sensory images and in discharging impulses to the muscular system. However, the area in one hemisphere seems to lead the other, or to trigger the other, in releasing nervous impulses and is therefore regarded as being the dominant one. With our earlier knowledge that each hemisphere controls the functions of the opposite side of the body we now can associate a dominant left hemisphere with a right-sided person and a dominant right hemisphere with a left-sided person. The dominant hemisphere also contains the control center for the language process: speaking, reading, and writing.

Ill Effects of Crossed Dominance

"All that is very interesting," parents have said, "but what will happen if I permit, or encourage, or force my left-eyed child to write with his right hand?" A study of the relation of eye and hand dominance reveals that not one single claim has been made of personal and physiological benefits to the child from such a course of action. On the other hand, there is evidence of adverse effects in many cases.

Numerous studies have been made of the relation of reading, writing, and speech problems to eye and hand dominance. Some authorities believe that the "confusion of cerebral dominance" resulting when the left-eyed child becomes right handed is the cause of some of the difficulties in reading and writing, characterized by reversals of letters and groups of letters.

Dr. Margaret M. Clark, in her book, *Left Handedness*, says, "Many of these crossed dominant children are found in the category of bad writers."[1] At California State Polytechnic College in San Luis Obispo, all freshman take a battery of guidance tests including measures for rate of reading, rate of writing, and a ten minute rapid theme writing on a fanciful topic. Crossed dominant students read more slowly and produce more erratic, illegible writing.

What is probably the largest sampling of eye dominance ever made is that done by the Human Engineering Laboratory in connection with its administration of an aptitude test battery to more than four hundred thousand students and adults since 1922. C. V. Broadley and M. E. Broadley in their book, *Know Your Real Abilities*, discuss the research work of this nation-wide organization on the relation of eye and hand dominance to personal, educational, and voca-

---

[1]M. M. Clark, *Left Handedness*, (London: University of London Press, 1957).

tional problems.[2] The human engineers confirm the findings of educators and medical scientists that approximately one quarter of the population is left eyed.

In one study of fifteen-year-old Chicago boys, the Laboratory found in the left-eyed, left-handed group no noticeable speech irregularities, unnatural nervousness, or serious reading difficulties. Among the group who were left eyed but right handed, it found forty-three percent of the boys suffering from extreme nervousness and with speech and reading abnormalities.

The Laboratory's policy of giving the same basic battery of tests to everyone, and the practice of many entire families asking to be tested, have made it possible for research studies to be made on the inheritance of eye dominance and the various aptitudes.

Changing to the Left Hand

"Training my baby to be left handed will be easy," said one mother. "My real worry is what to do with my nine-year-old son who is left eyed but right handed." The conservative answer to this question would be to make a gradual change to the left hand only on the evidence of tension, nervousness, chewing of finger nails, or other nervous behavior.

However, the ill effects of crossed dominance do not always appear as early as childhood. Some students work off their nervous energy in physical activities and experience the tension of crossed dominance for the first time when they settle down in some sedentary occupation. Others, through either luck or some inner urge, go into physically active occupations and escape any serious effects until retirement. Some men and women past retirement age, though apparently suffering no abnormal results of crossed dominance, are compulsively engaged in some physical activity, always on the go. Because of the possible delayed ill effects of crossed dominance, parents should not wait for nervousness and tension to appear before encouraging a crossed dominant child to use the left hand.

However, it is never too late to change. Broadley and Broadley tell of a moderately successful Boston lawyer who was tested at the age of fifty-seven. He scored in aptitudes as a perfect lawyer and had an extensive vocabulary, but suffered from stammering. On learning that he was left eyed, he decided to make himself left handed gradually. Three years later he reported that his stammering had stopped. It must be noted that crossed dominance is only one of a number of causes of speech difficulties.

THE TASK OF CHANGING to the left hand is easier for children. An ideal situation is one in which a left-eyed parent and the child together make of it a stunt or game, starting with a simple thing like holding a drinking glass, gradually adding other easy activities, and making a habit of each one before attempting another. Changing the handwriting to the left hand should come last in cases where handwriting skill is already established. Changing the writing hand must

---

[2]C. V. Broadley and M. E. Broadley, *Know Your Real Abilities,* (New York: McGraw Hill, 1948).

be done gradually. Start out by learning to sign your name. Blackboard writing or large crayon writing on paper might be a wise step.

The important thing in the whole process of changing over is for you to accept yourself as a left-sided person. As with many crossed dominants, the new concept of yourself as being left sided may dispel a mental fog, previously felt but never understood.

Left handedness in these modern times, in addition to being justified on a scientific basis, is becoming more socially acceptable. There was a time, not so very long ago, when the left-handed person was considered to be possessed by evil spirits. The very word for left, sinister, also has meant: dishonest, unlucky, bad. Religion has regarded right and left in the same manner. The good sheep in the parable are assembled on the right, the wicked goats on the left. Dante's downward path in the Inferno is always to the left, but his ascent in Purgatory is by the right. The Eight-Fold Way of Buddhism towards Nirvana is always to the right. Similarly the Apostles' Creed states that Christ sits on the right hand of God, and the pious Mohammedan makes a point of entering a mosque with his right foot first. The same attitude is found in politics, where the opposition party sits on the left. Even the modern business executive speaks of his right hand man.

A few parents cling to the old superstitious beliefs and occasionally we find a teacher still dedicated to making this a world of right handers. Fortunately, most educators now follow the practice of permitting each child to write with his preferred hand. Permissiveness, however, on the part of the parents and teachers is not enough. Left-sided children continue to imitate the right-handed majority and yield to the hidden social pressures to conform. The next step for society to take is to remove these pressures. The next step for educators, already taken by a few, is to measure the eye dominance of each child as he enters school for the first time and to encourage the use of his corresponding hand in writing and in other skills. The next step for parents is to accurately determine and deliberately train their left-sided children.

Southpaws in School

An exclusive Southpaw Club was organized in a West Texas school several years ago with a membership of over 40, limited to left handers and to the rookies who were just beginning to use the left hand. They pooled their ideas and experiences. By sitting on the right side of the classroom their eagle eyes could keep watch on the teacher and the common kids.

By sitting on the left side of study halls, where there were no distractions on the side of their dominant eyes, they found that they could concentrate better. They used ball point pens, soft pencils, and hard paper to make easier the job of handwriting. They all learned to use the typewriter after one of their members read somewhere that the letters made by the fingers of the left hand are used more often than the letters made by the right. In the following year several members of the club won prizes for their typing speed.

Those who joined the school orchestra or band chose the French horn, designed for left hand fingering, or instruments that use both hands, such as the clarinet, saxophone, drums, or one of the stringed instruments. Those who studied piano found that their left hand playing was commended.

By shopping and by correspondence they discovered that manufacturers are making more and more things for southpaws: scissors, metal shears, fishing rods, golf clubs, baseball gloves, bowling balls, rifles, shotguns, potato peelers, apple corers, can openers, ironing boards, irons, pencil sharpeners, desk arm chairs, dental instruments, refrigerators, artist palettes, lettering pens, and drafting machines. They persuaded a local bank to furnish left-handed checkbooks, with the stub at the right.

The boys organized a baseball team and challenged the right wingers. A number of the players developed into first rate switch hitters.

The whole club, by their own initiative and cooperative effort, converted what had been a minority with a liability into an accepted and respected group. As a result, the increased self confidence of each member helped him to find his right place in the world where society ultimately will accept him as one of her own.

About the Authors . . .

NORMA BANAS is curriculum consultant at Educational Guidance Services, Miami, Florida. In addition to her work in designing educational and remedial approaches for children with reading and learning problems, Mrs. Banas is a contributing editor to Academic Therapy.

JOAN CARTER is instructional materials specialist in a school for physically and mentally handicapped children, Los Angeles, California. She formerly was a teacher of the learning disabled, and has trained teachers for work in this field.

BEN CROUTCH is assistant superintendent of special services and special schools for Imperial County, California. His background includes teaching at all levels, and work in the field of learning disabilities. At the present time, he supervises a number of special programs.

GEORGE EARLY is clinical director, Achievement Center for Children, Purdue University, West Lafayette, Indiana. Mr. Early's works appear in the Charles E. Merrill Slow Learners Series. In addition, he is a contributing editor to Academic Therapy.

DORIS C. ENSTROM is director of training and consultant services for Peterson Handwriting, Greensburg, Pennsylvania. Long active in the field, Mrs. Enstrom wrote the script for the MacMillan Adventures in Handwriting series and for the Peterson Handwriting Teacher's Guide and Pupils' Kits.

E. A. ENSTROM, Ph.D., is director of research and instructional development, Peterson Handwriting, Greensburg, Pennsylvania. Dr. Enstrom lectures extensively, is involved in continuing research, and has published a number of papers in the professional literature.

EDITH FISHER has been an active member of the Canadian Association for Children with Learning Disabilities, Toronto, Canada, in which she has served as publications chairman.

ENID M. HARRISON is senior teacher, Forest Town School for Cerebral Palsied Children, Johannesburg, South Africa. For the past seventeen years, Mrs. Harrison has taught children with special learning needs. She is also a correspondent to Academic Therapy.

EARL J. HEATH, Ph.D., is chairman, special education section, department of education, and executive director, Achievement Center for Children, Purdue University, West Lafayette, Indiana. He has been active in learning disabilities for a number of years.

HAROLD B. HELMS has a background in both regular and special education. In addition, he has experience in educational therapy with the learning disabled. He is currently doing advanced graduate work in remedial education.

RUTH IOGHA was formerly a member of the faculty, Kaliski School, New York City, where, from 1959 to 1969, she was both director of music and educational coordinator. Mrs. Iogha is now a member of the music department faculty, State University College, Potsdam, New York.

ERNEST J. KAHN, O.D. maintains his private practice in optometry in Walpole, Massachusetts. An active lecturer and worker in the field of visual problems in children, Dr. Kahn is chairman of the committee on visual training, Massachusetts Society of Optometrists.

LOTTE KALISKI is founder and director emerita, The Kaliski Schools, New York and New Jersey. After many years in the field, Miss Kaliski now serves as chief consultant to the schools, assisting in the development of curriculum, special remedial methods, training, and programing.

GERALDINE M. KIMMELL has been coordinating editor of Academic Therapy since its founding in 1965. In addition, Mrs. Kimmell is curriculum coordinator of prescribed techniques, DeWitt Reading Clinic, San Rafael, California. She is also co-author, Screening Test for Auditory Perception Academic Therapy Publications, San Rafael, Ca.).

DIANA HANBURY KING, M.A. Honors, has been director for fifteen years of both The Kildonan School, Solebury, Pennsylvania, and Dunnabeck, a summer camp, Farmington, Pennsylvania. Both facilities offer programs designed specifically to meet the needs of the dyslexic student.

CHARLOTTE E. LARSON is assistant director of special education, Joliet, Illinois, public schools. Following a background of work with Dr. A. A. Strauss and Dr. L. E. Lehtinen, Miss Larson started the first classes in a public school in the United States for brain-injured children.

NORMAN LEVINE is director, Leila Armstrong Reading Clinic, Downey, California. Mr. Levine's background includes work in the regular classroom and in remedial settings. He is currently the principal of a school for physically and mentally handicapped children, Los Angeles, California.

SHIRLEY LINN is a teacher in the Auburn Washburn Unified School District 437, Topeka, Kansas. Mrs. Linn's experiences in education include teaching the neurologically impaired, homebound children, and kindergarten classes. She has also taught teacher training classes at the college level.

LAWRENCE W. MACDONALD, O.D., maintains his private practice in optometry in Newton, Massachusetts. At present Dr. Macdonald is studying the relationship of visual deficiencies to flicker fusion. A member of several organizations, Dr. Macdonald has published in professional publications.

BETTY D. MADISON teaches educationally handicapped children in the public schools of Lafayette, California. In addition to her work in regular elementary and preschool education, Mrs. Madison has held a number of consultancies, and master teaching responsibilities. She has also published in the field.

ALICE R. McKENNA is director of evaluation, DeWitt Reading Clinic, San Rafael, California. She is an experienced teacher whose background includes classroom teaching, kindergarten through college levels, remedial teaching, the instruction of handicapped children, and the training of teachers.

CHRISTINE McMONAGLE is an active worker in the field of learning disabled children. She has been associated with the Canadian Association for Children with Learning Disabilities, Toronto, Canada, in which she has served as acting executive director.

HARRIS L. PREFONTAINE, O.D., is an optometrist in Grand Rapids, Michigan. Dr. PreFontaine has held a number of positions with various professional organizations. A fellow of the American Academy of Optometry, Dr. PreFontaine has served as a consultant to several Michigan school districts.

JESSIE RAMMING is director of the private elementary school that bears her name, located in Lompoc, California, and which she has operated for the past twelve years. Prior to this, Mrs. Ramming had extensive experience with children in multigraded rural schools.

RANDY RAMOS is in his second year of college, graduating from the public school system in California. Prior to his graduation, Mr. Ramos received special assistance in the language areas from a private tutor.

MARTHA SERIO is teacher-consultant to the programs for neurologically handicapped children, Columbus, Ohio, public schools. Mrs. Serio has a broad range of educational experiences, has written for the professional literature, and has lectured at the college level. She is also a contributing editor to Academic Therapy.

ALETHA P. THOMAS has been a teacher of educationally handicapped children, Alameda, California, City Schools, for the past twelve years. Prior to this, Miss Thomas taught the mentally retarded, supervised programs for the orthopedically handicapped, and taught in the regular classroom.

DEAN TREMBLY, Ed.D. is test officer and counselor at the Counseling and Testing Center, California State Polytechnic College, San Luis Obispo, California. Dr. Trembly, in addition to an extensive background in public school and college teaching, serves as a consultant to several industrial firms.

I. H. WILLS is diagnostic counselor, Educational Guidance Services, Miami, Florida. Prior to her work in developing remedial programs for children with special learning disabilities, Mrs. Wills did social work with children and adults. She is also a contributing editor to Academic Therapy.